Practising Evidence-based
CHILD HEALTH

Maud Meates FRCPCH
Olivier Duperrex MD
Ruth Gilbert MD
Stuart Logan FRCPCH

At the Centre for Evidence-based Child Health
Institute of Child Health, London

Editor
Sharon E Straus

At the NHS R&D Centre for Evidence-based Medicine
Nuffield Department of Clinical Medicine
Level 5, John Radcliffe Hospital
Headley Way, Headington
Oxford OX3 9DU

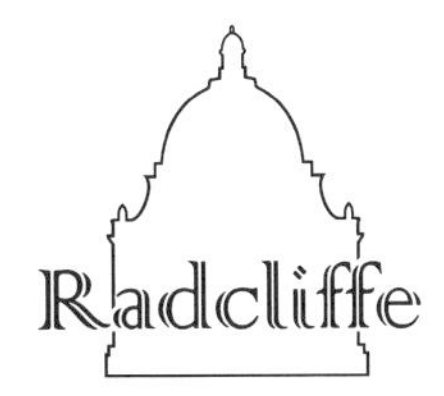

Radcliffe Medical Press
18 Marcham Road, Abingdon, Oxon OX14 1AA, UK
Tel: 01235 528820 Fax: 01235 528830
e-mail: medical@radpress.win-uk.net

Radcliffe Medical Press Ltd
18 Marcham Road, Abingdon, Oxon OX14 1AA

British Library Cataloguing in Publication Data

A catalogue record for this book is available from the British Library.

ISBN 1 85775 410 7

Typeset by Advance Typesetting Ltd, Oxfordshire
Printed and bound in Great Britain by
TJ International Ltd, Padstow, Cornwall

CONTENTS

ACKNOWLEDGEMENTS

Radcliffe Medical Press acknowledges with gratitude the kind permission granted by publishers of the citation references for the full papers to be reproduced at the beginning of each session. These permissions prohibit further reproduction by photocopying or by electronic means and if this facility is required, further permission should be obtained from the source quoted in each case.

We are grateful to Sarah See at the Centre for Evidence-based Child Health for her help in compiling this manual.

Extracts from *Evidence-based Medicine: how to practice and teach EBM* (David Sackett *et al.*) which appear at the back of this manual are reproduced with the kind permission of Harcourt Brace & Co Ltd.

INTRODUCTION

This is a syllabus for a 7 session course for clinicians on how to practise evidence-based child health: that is, how to integrate our individual clinical expertise with a critical appraisal of the best available external clinical evidence from systematic research.

We see the practice of evidence-based medicine as a process of life-long, self-directed, problem-based learning in which caring for one's own patients creates the need for clinically important information about diagnosis, prognosis, therapy, and other clinical and healthcare issues, in which its practitioners:

1 convert these information needs into answerable questions;
2 track down, with maximum efficiency, the best evidence with which to answer them (making best use of the increasing variety of sources of primary and secondary evidence);
3 critically appraise that evidence for its validity (closeness to the truth), importance (size of effect) and usefulness (clinical applicability);
4 integrate the appraisal with clinical expertise and apply the results in clinical practice; and
5 evaluate their own performance.

This syllabus is designed to help clinicians develop and improve those skills.

Each of its 7 sessions is divided into 2 parts:

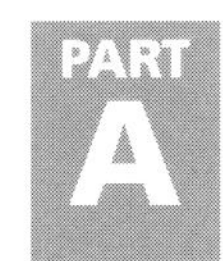

Part A: Going through the 5 steps with a patient, focusing on step 3 (critical appraisal), step 4 (integration with clinical expertise), and step 5 (self-evaluation).

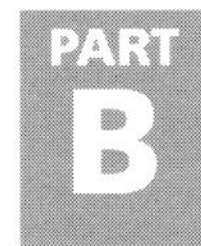

Part B: Skills training, focusing on step 1 (forming answerable clinical questions) and step 2 (finding the best evidence), in which we introduce a variety of sources of evidence plus some strategies for analysing, summarising and storing the evidence in the form of one-page summaries ('Critically Appraised Topics' or CATs).

Evidence-based Medicine: what it is and what it isn't

This is the text of an editorial from the *British Medical Journal* on 13th January 1996 (*BMJ* 1996; **312:** 71–2)

Authors:

David L Sackett, Professor, NHS Research and Development Centre for Evidence-based Medicine, Oxford.

William MC Rosenberg, Clinical Tutor in Medicine, Nuffield Department of Clinical Medicine, Oxford.

JA Muir Gray, Director of Research and Development, Anglia and Oxford Regional Health Authority, Milton Keynes.

R Brian Haynes, Professor of Medicine and Clinical Epidemiology, McMaster University Hamilton, Canada.

W Scott Richardson, Rochester, USA.

Evidence-based Medicine, whose philosophical origins extend back to mid-19th century Paris and earlier, remains a hot topic for clinicians, public health practitioners, purchasers, planners, and the public. There are now frequent workshops in how to practice and teach it (one sponsored by this journal will be held in London on April 24th); undergraduate [1] and post-graduate training programmes [2] are incorporating it [3] (or pondering how to do so); British centres for evidence-based practice have been established or planned in adult medicine, child health, surgery, pathology, pharmacotherapy, nursing, general practice, and dentistry; the Cochrane Collaboration and the York Centre for Review and Dissemination in York are providing systematic reviews of the effects of health care; new evidence-based practice journals are being launched; and it has become a common topic in the lay media. But enthusiasm has been mixed with some negative reaction [4–6]. Criticism has ranged from evidence-based medicine being old-hat to it being a dangerous innovation, perpetrated by the arrogant to serve cost-cutters and suppress clinical freedom. As evidence-based medicine continues to evolve and adapt, now is a useful time to refine the discussion of what it is and what it is not.

Evidence-based medicine is the conscientious, explicit and judicious use of current best evidence in making decisions about the care of individual patients. The practice of evidence-based medicine means integrating individual clinical expertise with the best available external clinical evidence from systematic research. By individual clinical expertise we mean the proficiency and judgement that individual clinicians acquire through clinical experience and clinical practice. Increased expertise is reflected in many ways, but especially in more effective and efficient diagnosis and in the more thoughtful identification and compassionate use of individual patients' predicaments, rights, and preferences in making clinical decisions about their care. By best available external clinical evidence we mean clinically relevant research, often from the basic sciences of medicine, but especially from patient centred clinical research into the accuracy and precision of diagnostic tests (including the clinical examination), the power of prognostic markers, and the efficacy and safety of therapeutic, rehabilitative, and preventive regimens. External clinical evidence both invalidates previously accepted diagnostic tests and treatments and replaces them with new ones that are more powerful, more accurate, more efficacious, and safer.

Good doctors use both individual clinical expertise and the best available external evidence, and neither alone is enough. Without clinical expertise, practice risks becoming tyrannised by evidence, for even excellent external evidence may be inapplicable to or inappropriate for an individual patient. Without current best evidence, practice risks becoming rapidly out of date, to the detriment of patients.

This description of what evidence-based medicine is helps clarify what evidence-based medicine is not. Evidence-based medicine is neither old-hat nor impossible to practice. The argument that everyone already is doing it falls before evidence of striking variations in both the integration of patient values into our clinical behaviour [7] and in the rates with which clinicians provide interventions to their patients [8]. The difficulties that clinicians face in keeping abreast of all the medical advances reported in primary journals are obvious from a comparison of the time required for reading (for general medicine, enough to examine

19 articles per day, 365 days per year [9]) with the time available (well under an hour per week by British medical consultants, even on self-reports [10]).

The argument that evidence-based medicine can be conducted only from ivory towers and armchairs is refuted by audits in the front lines of clinical care where at least some inpatient clinical teams in general medicine [11], psychiatry (JR Geddes *et al.*, Royal College of Psychiatrists winter meeting, January 1996), and surgery (P McCulloch, personal communication) have provided evidence-based care to the vast majority of their patients. Such studies show that busy clinicians who devote their scarce reading time to selective, efficient, patient-driven searching, appraisal and incorporation of the best available evidence can practice evidence-based medicine.

Evidence-based medicine is not 'cook-book' medicine. Because it requires a bottom-up approach that integrates the best external evidence with individual clinical expertise and patient-choice, it cannot result in slavish, cook-book approaches to individual patient care. External clinical evidence can inform, but can never replace, individual clinical expertise, and it is this expertise that decides whether the external evidence applies to the individual patient at all and, if so, how it should be integrated into a clinical decision. Similarly, any external guideline must be integrated with individual clinical expertise in deciding whether and how it matches the patient's clinical state, predicament, and preferences, and thus whether it should be applied. Clinicians who fear top-down cook-books will find the advocates of evidence-based medicine joining them at the barricades.

Evidence-based medicine is not cost-cutting medicine. Some fear that evidence-based medicine will be hijacked by purchasers and managers to cut the costs of health care. This would not only be a misuse of evidence-based medicine but suggests a fundamental misunderstanding of its financial consequences. Doctors practising evidence-based medicine will identify and apply the most efficacious interventions to maximise the quality and quantity of life for individual patients; this may raise rather than lower the cost of their care.

Evidence-based medicine is not restricted to randomised trials and meta-analyses. It involves tracking down the best external evidence with which to answer our clinical questions. To find out about the accuracy of a diagnostic test, we need to find proper cross-sectional studies of patients clinically suspected of harbouring the relevant disorder, not a randomised trial. For a question about prognosis, we need proper follow-up studies of patients assembled at a uniform, early point in the clinical course of their disease. And sometimes the evidence we need will come from the basic sciences such as genetics or immunology. It is when asking questions about therapy that we should try to avoid the non-experimental approaches, since these routinely lead to false-positive conclusions about efficacy. Because the randomised trial, and especially the systematic review of several randomised trials, is so much more likely to inform us and so much less likely to mislead us, it has become the 'gold standard' for judging whether a treatment does more good than harm. However, some questions about therapy do not require randomised trials (successful interventions for otherwise fatal conditions) or cannot wait for the trials to be conducted. And if no randomised trial has been carried out for our patient's predicament, we follow the trail to the next best external evidence and work from there.

Despite its ancient origins, evidence-based medicine remains a relatively young discipline whose positive impacts are just beginning to be validated [12, 13], and it will continue to evolve. This evolution will be enhanced as several undergraduate, post-graduate, and continuing medical education programmes adopt and adapt it to their learners' needs. These programmes, and their evaluation, will provide further information and understanding about what evidence-based medicine is, and what it is not.

References

1 British Medical Association: *Report of the working party on medical education*. London: British Medical Association, 1995.

2 Standing Committee on Postgraduate Medical and Dental Education: *Creating a better learning environment in hospitals: 1 Teaching hospital doctors and dentists to teach*. London: SCOPME, 1994.

3 General Medical Council: *Education Committee Report*. London: General Medical Council, 1994.

4 Grahame-Smith D: Evidence-based medicine: Socratic dissent. *BMJ* 1995; 310: 1126–7.

5 Evidence-based medicine, in its place (editorial). *Lancet* 1995; 346: 785.

6 Correspondence. Evidence-based Medicine. *Lancet* 1995; 346: 1171–2.

7 Weatherall DJ: The inhumanity of medicine. *BMJ* 1994; 308: 1671–2.

8 House of Commons Health Committee. *Priority setting in the NHS: purchasing*. First report sessions 1994–95. London: HMSO, 1995, (HC 134–1).

9 Davidoff F, Haynes B, Sackett D, Smith R: Evidence-based medicine; a new journal to help doctors identify the information they need. *BMJ* 1995; 310: 1085–6.

10 Sackett DL: Surveys of self-reported reading times of consultants in Oxford, Birmingham, Milton-Keynes, Bristol, Leicester, and Glasgow, 1995. In Rosenberg WMC, Richardson WS, Haynes RB, Sackett DL. *Evidence-based Medicine*. London: Churchill-Livingstone, 1999.

11 Ellis J, Mulligan I, Rowe J, Sackett DL: Inpatient general medicine is evidence based. *Lancet* 1995; 346: 407–10.

12 Bennett RJ, Sackett DL, Haynes RB, Neufeld VR: A controlled trial of teaching critical appraisal of the clinical literature to medical students. *JAMA* 1987; 257: 2451–4.

13 Shin JH, Haynes RB, Johnston ME: Effect of problem-based, self-directed undergraduate education on life-long learning. *Can Med Assoc J* 1993; 148: 969–76.

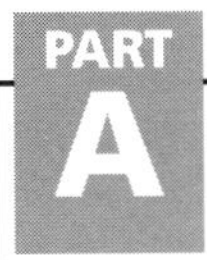

Critical appraisal of a clinical article about therapy

EBCH SESSION

1

SECTION 1

Therapy and introduction to CATS

Section 1: Nurse-led asthma training

A nurse on the children's ward, where you are the nursing manager of the paediatric service, comes to you expressing concern at the high number of children readmitted with asthma. (Asthma is the commonest diagnosis at discharge in your service.) The nurse has just finished a diploma in asthma and believes that you should consider creating a paediatric asthma nurse specialist post. She believes that such a person would be able to offer education and support to families and children after discharge, and would have an impact on readmission rates. A recent audit of your service reveals you have an 18% readmissions rate. She presents you with a search strategy and a research article.

You have scarce resources, but are aware of the large number of admissions and readmissions with asthma, and the cost of this for the service. You must consider whether creating such a post would be likely to have enough of an effect to cover the implementation costs. You formulate the question, in children hospitalised for asthma, can a nurse-led home asthma management programme decrease readmission for asthma?

Search strategy for nurse-led asthma training

Type in:
1 explode "ASTHMA"/ all subheadings
2 explode "CHILD"/ all subheadings
3 explode "PATIENT-READMISSION"/ all subheadings
4 #1 and #2 and #3
5 PT = "RANDOMIZED-CONTROLLED-TRIAL"
6 #4 and #5

You find the article by Madge *et al.* (*Thorax* 1997; **52:** 223–8)

Read this article and decide:
1 Is the evidence from this randomised trial valid?
2 If valid, is this evidence important?
3 If valid and important, can you apply this evidence in caring for your patient(s)?

If you want to read some strategies for answering these sorts of questions, you could have a look at pp 91–6, 133–41 and 166–72 in *Evidence-based Medicine*.

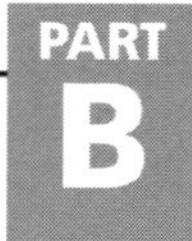

How to use the CATMaker software (optional)

If a CATMaker is provided with this package you will be shown how to use it to generate and save your own one page 'critically appraised topic' (CAT) from an article about therapy. The advantages of the CATMaker include its ability to calculate for you the clinically useful measures of the effects of therapy and their confidence intervals, and to save your critical appraisal for printing, sharing and storage.

Impact of a nurse-led home management training programme in children admitted to hospital with acute asthma: a randomised controlled study

Philippa Madge, John McColl, James Paton

Abstract

Background – Re-admissions to hospital in childhood asthma are common with studies reporting that 25% or more of children will be re-admitted within a year. There is a need for strategies to reduce re-admissions.

Methods – A prospective randomised control study of an asthma home management training programme was performed in children aged two years or over admitted with acute asthma. Two hundred and one children were randomised at admission to either an intervention group (n = 96) which received the teaching programme or a control group (n = 105). A nurse-led teaching programme used the current attack as a model for the management of future attacks and included discussion, written information, subsequent follow up and telephone advice aimed at developing and reinforcing individualised asthma management plans. Parents were also provided with a course of oral steroids and guidance on when to start them.

Results – The groups were similar in degree of social deprivation, length of stay, number of previous admissions, acute asthma treatment, and asthma treatment at discharge. Subsequent re-admissions were significantly reduced in the intervention group from 25% to 8% in individual follow up periods that ranged from two to 14 months ($\chi^2 = 9.63$; $p = 0.002$). This reduction was not accompanied by any increase in subsequent emergency room attendances nor, in the short term, by any increase in urgent community asthma treatment. The intervention group also showed significant reductions in day and night morbidity 3–4 weeks after admission to hospital.

Conclusions – A nurse-led asthma home management training programme administered during a hospital admission can significantly reduce subsequent admissions to hospital for asthma. Acute hospitalisation may be a particularly effective time to deliver home management training.

(*Thorax* 1997;52:223–228)

Keywords: children, asthma, self-management.

Department of Child Health, Royal Hospital for Sick Children, Yorkhill NHS Trust, Glasgow G3 8SJ, UK
P Madge
J Paton

Department of Statistics, University of Glasgow, Glasgow, UK
J McColl

Correspondence to:
Dr J Y Paton.

Received 1 August 1996
Returned to authors 2 October 1996
Revised version received 1 November 1996
Accepted for publication 20 November 1996

Over the last two decades there has been a dramatic rise in admissions to hospital for childhood asthma.[1,2] Asthma re-admissions are also common. For example, Senthilsevan recently reported that re-admission rates (asthma re-admissions/all asthma admissions) for children from all 134 hospitals in Saskatchewan Province, Canada were between 20% and 30% during the decade 1980–9.[3] Mitchell *et al* reported higher rates in children in New Zealand[4] and there is even some evidence that re-admissions may be increasing.[5] The need to develop strategies to reduce the high re-admission rate in childhood asthma has been highlighted.[4]

At the Royal Hospital for Sick Children, Glasgow we also noted that asthma re-admissions were common with approximately 21% of children being re-admitted within a year. This occurred despite the fact that over 90% of the children admitted to hospital received nebulised bronchodilators and oral corticosteroids. Care around discharge was, however, less satisfactory – for example, only 10% were noted to have been given written instructions about their treatment.

There are now many published studies on the use of asthma self-management programmes to decrease asthma morbidity. Several narrative reviews have evaluated the existing paediatric literature and found positive results for some programmes and inconclusive results for others.[6–9] Howland *et al* commented that many of the studies do not stand up to rigorous scientific scrutiny.[8] Limitations included small sample sizes, lack of a control group, and a reliance on a select population of volunteers. There was also substantial variation in the asthma education programmes used and their duration. A more recently published meta-analysis of home management training programmes in children with asthma confined to randomised control trials of adequate quality also concluded that such programmes did not seem to reduce morbidity.[10] This analysis concluded by suggesting that teaching programmes designed for targeted audiences with well defined characteristics such as disease severity might be more likely to show benefits.

In an attempt to reduce our high asthma re-admission rate and to address deficiencies in discharge care we planned to introduce a nurse-led home management training programme. We specifically hypothesised that such a training programme delivered during an admission for acute asthma would reduce subsequent re-admissions. However, such an approach is expensive to implement and, as the above evidence summarises, has not unequivocally decreased morbidity. To evaluate its impact on morbidity and provide evidence for its continued use we therefore introduced the programme as a randomised control study. This report describes the observed outcomes.

Methods

SUBJECTS

The study was performed in the four medical wards of the Royal Hospital for Sick Children, Glasgow, a large children's hospital providing care for a population of approximately 173 000 children under 14 years of age in the Greater Glasgow Health Board Area in the West of Scotland.

All children over two years of age admitted with acute asthma between January 1994 and January 1995 were eligible. Children under two years with acute wheezing were excluded for two reasons – firstly, because bronchiolitis, an acute wheezing illness which occurs mainly in children under two years and is caused by a viral infection, is difficult to distinguish from asthma, and secondly, because there is less agreement about the nature and diagnosis of asthma in young children under two years of age.[11]

The study was reviewed and approved by the ethics committee of the Royal Hospital for Sick Children. It was their view that the proposed nurse-led training programme addressed an identified clinical deficiency and that the randomised introduction did not require informed consent. Accordingly, detailed written informed consent was not sought from either group before randomisation or, in the intervention group, before the training programme which was introduced as usual care. After verbal explanation no children or parents refused to receive the home management training. For both the groups ("intervention" and "control" or usual care) all clinical care, including decisions about drug management and medical follow up, were determined by their attending paediatrician following standard practice. Parents within the control group were not aware that other children were receiving the educational intervention nor that subsequent admissions were being tracked.

RANDOMISATION

Randomisation was performed before the study by drawing cards and allocating each sequential future admission to either an intervention or a control group. Eligible children with acute asthma were then entered at admission into the pre-assigned groups. In order to standardise the intervention for each child in the intervention group children had to be identified and families contacted within 24 hours of admission. This was not always practical, particularly at weekends when the nurse was not available. The solution adopted was to recruit only on Monday to Friday when the asthma nurse (PM) was available. To monitor for any resulting selection bias, clinical information – including details of hospital re-admissions and re-attendances – on all children eligible but not randomised was collected retrospectively. The study was not confined to children having their first ever admission for asthma and included children with a varying number of previous admissions (table 1). However, children were eligible for randomisation only on the first admission with acute asthma during the study year.

INTERVENTION

For the study a structured asthma education and home management training programme was developed. In order to minimise variations in its delivery the package was implemented by one trained specialist asthma nurse (PM). The package consisted of review discussion sessions, written information and advice, and subsequent follow up and telephone advice.

Review discussion sessions

The study nurse briefly met all parents within 24 hours of admission and then had, on average, two further longer teaching/discussion sessions with each family, amounting in total to about 45 minutes.

Written information and advice

At the first meeting each family was given a highly visual "Going home with asthma" booklet developed specifically to provide basic practical advice about asthma. The booklet included chapters about the nature of asthma, its triggers, and its treatment including the use and side effects of corticosteroids. It also described signs commonly present in impending asthma attacks[12] and encouraged parents to recognise such signs in their own children. The booklet was used as the focus of discussion in the two subsequent meetings. In particular, the symptoms and signs identified by the parent as preceding the child's present attack were used as the basis of an individualised symptom based asthma management plan. Parents of children over five were also provided with a peak flow meter and instructed about flow monitoring. They were free to choose whether they preferred a plan based on peak flow measurements or symptoms, or both.

A written summary of the agreed management plan was provided for each family on a credit card sized card.[13] Each family was also provided with a course of oral steroids with guidance on when to start them.

Subsequent follow up and telephone advice

All children in the intervention group were given one appointment 2–3 weeks after discharge for a nurse-run asthma clinic where the previous advice and home management plan were reviewed and reinforced. Throughout the study telephone advice from the nurse was available to the study group about aspects of chronic management.

Table 1 Characteristics of the study groups and their inpatient asthma care

	Intervention group (n = 96)	*Control group (n = 105)*	*Non-randomised group (n = 82)*
M:F	62:34 (1.82:1)	62:43 (1.44:1)	51:31 (1.64:1)
Age			
2–5 years	40 (41.7%)	53 (55.2%)	42 (51.2%)
5–10 years	41 (42.7%)	25 (23.8%)	32 (39.0%)
>10 years	15 (15.6%)	22 (21.0%)	8 (9.8%)
Median (range) age (years)	6.0 (2.0–13.1)	4.23 (2.0–15.3)	4.93 (2.1–13.4)
Median (range) deprivation score*	5.5 (1–7)	6.0 (1–7)	5 (1–7)
Median (range) length of stay (days)	2 (1–11)	2 (1–13)	2 (0–9)
Median (range) number of previous admissions	2 (0–8)	2 (0–19)	2 (0–8)
Median (range) days follow up	210 (63–428)	209 (64–428)	254 (64–432)
Nebulised bronchodilator	96 (100%)	104 (99.0%)	82 (100%)
Oral steroids	93 (96.9%)	101 (96.2%)	79 (96.3%)
Oxygen therapy	38 (39.6%)	39 (37.1%)	28 (34.1%)
Intravenous aminophylline	8 (8.3%)	10 (9.5%)	9 (11.0%)

* Deprivation score based on postcode[15]: 1 = least deprived, 7 = most deprived.

OUTCOMES

Primary outcome: subsequent admissions to hospital

The principal focus of this study was the impact of the home management training programme on asthma re-admissions so the primary outcome was the number of subsequent admissions to hospital with acute asthma. All hospital admissions for acute asthma were monitored during the study allowing any child who was re-admitted to be identified. A re-admission was defined as any child who had a subsequent asthma admission after an index admission during the study period of 14 months. Decisions to admit were made by the clinical staff in the emergency room who had no information on whether the child had been in the intervention or control group.

Secondary outcomes

(1) Subsequent attendances at the emergency room: after an index admission any subsequent attendance at the hospital emergency room during the study period was also noted.

(2) Asthma morbidity: a morbidity questionnaire (based on the index of perceived symptoms developed by Usherwood[14]) to assess asthma symptoms was sent to families in both groups four weeks after discharge from hospital. This instrument gives three scores for asthma morbidity: day disturbance, night disturbance, and disability. An additional question on attendance at the family practitioner for urgent asthma treatment in the period following discharge was also included.

DATA ANALYSIS

Data were summarised using standard descriptive statistics (mean and standard deviation for continuous data, median and range for discrete data). Hypotheses about proportions were tested using χ^2. Medians were compared using the Mann-Whitney U test. Subsequent admissions to hospital were analysed using statistical techniques for the analysis of survival data, principally Cox's proportional hazard model. p values of less than 0.05 were considered significant.

All analyses were performed on an IBM compatible computer using Minitab vs 8 or SPSS for Windows.

Table 2 Comparison between control and intervention groups of asthma treatment before admission, and asthma treatment and follow up arranged during the index admission

	Intervention group (n = 96)	*Control group (n = 105)*	*p value*
Bronchodilators before admission	77 (80.2%)	97 (92.4%)	0.012
Bronchodilators after admission	96 (100%)	104 (99.0%)	NS
Inhaled prophylaxis before admission	47 (49.0%)	60 (57.1%)	NS
Inhaled prophylaxis after admission	76 (79.2%)	86 (81.9%)	NS
Review of inhaled device technique	94 (97.9%)	96 (91.4%)	0.044
Follow up hospital medical appointment	59 (61.5%)	80 (76.2%)	0.024

Results

Two hundred and eighty three children over two years of age with acute asthma were admitted of which 201 were randomised into the study, 96 into the intervention group and 105 into the control group. The intervention and control groups were similar in terms of median length of stay, median number of previous admissions, and acute asthma therapy. Information on socioeconomic deprivation, derived from post code,[15] was no different between the groups with both showing high levels of deprivation. The children randomised to the intervention group were slightly older at six years (table 1). Physician initiated asthma treatment is shown in table 2. At discharge there was no significant difference in the use of inhaled bronchodilator or prophylactic therapy. Use of devices was checked in over 90% of both groups, although slightly more frequently in the intervention group. In contrast, medical follow up was actually arranged more frequently in the control group.

Another 82 children (non-randomised group) would have been eligible for inclusion but were admitted on days when they could not be followed. Clinical details including inpatient hospital treatment for these children are also summarised in table 1. It can be seen that these children were very similar to the children in the two study groups. Outcome questionnaires were not completed by the non-randomised group and only data on re-admissions and re-attendances at the emergency room were available.

PRIMARY OUTCOME

Asthma re-admissions were monitored until two months after randomisation ended, a total

Table 3 Hospital re-admissions and emergency room re-attendances with acute asthma

	Intervention group	*Control group*	*Non-randomised group*
Re-admitted to hospital	8 (8.3)*	26 (24.8)	18 (22.0)
Re-attended hospital emergency room	7 (7.3)	7 (6.7)	8 (9.8)
Re-attended family practitioner**	11 (11.5)	7 (6.7)	N/A

Values in parentheses are percentages.
*χ^2=9.63; p=0.002 (intervention group versus control group).
**Re-attended family practitioner 3–4 weeks following discharge for urgent asthma treatment.

Table 5 Median (range) morbidity at 3–4 weeks after discharge as assessed by parent completed postal questionnaire

	Intervention group	*Control group*	*p value**
Day score	4.0 (0–16)	7.0 (0–16)	0.0005
Night score	4.0 (0–12)	6.0 (0–12)	0.0002
Disability score	4.0 (0–32)	8.0 (0–32)	0.078

*Mann-Whitney U test.

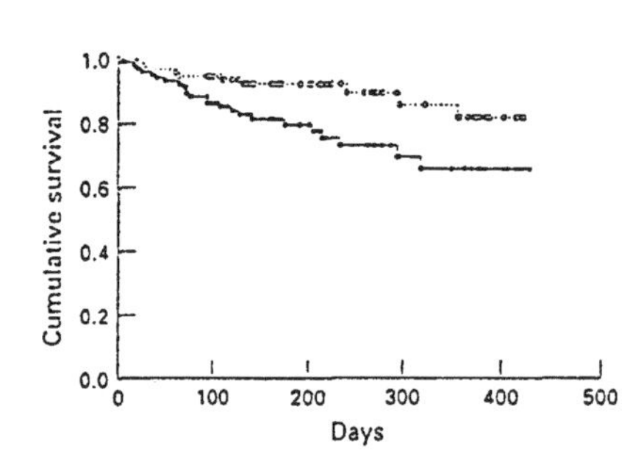

Figure 1 Cumulative survival curve showing time to re-admission for the intervention (O) and control (●) groups. Because the survival curve adjusts for the differing length of follow up, the percentages "surviving" (not re-admitted) are not directly applicable to table 3.

of 14 months in all, when the re-admission data were censored. This gave individual follow up periods of 2–14 months. A simple χ^2 test (table 3) indicated that the re-admission rate was significantly lower in the intervention group (8.3%) than in the control group (24.8%).

Survival analysis was then used to explore whether or not re-admission was influenced by group type (control versus intervention), number of previous asthma admissions, previous asthma drug therapy, oxygen saturation on admission, whether intravenous theophylline was used,[4] age, and sex (table 3, fig 1). An initial analysis using a log rank test examined the effect of each individual variable on survival. Group, number of previous admissions, and prophylactic asthma therapy were all significant. Applying Cox's proportional hazards model and entering explanatory variables in a stepwise manner from the full list of variables above, the only significant remaining factors were the number of previous admissions and group.

Randomisation resulted in a difference in age structure between groups with fewer younger children in the intervention group (table 1). Because of this, the Cox's proportional hazard analysis was repeated after stratifying for age. Both previous admissions and group remained significant ($p<0.0001$; $p=0.03$). Thus, the structured home management training programme remained significantly associated with a reduced risk of re-admission even after age had been accounted for (table 4).

SECONDARY OUTCOMES

Emergency room re-attendances

There was no difference in the number of emergency room attendances between the two groups nor any difference in re-attendance at the family practitioner in the 3–4 weeks following discharge for urgent asthma treatment (table 3).

Morbidity

Morbidity questionnaires were returned by 129 families (63 intervention group (65.6%) and 66 control group (62.9%)). Day, night, and disability scores were calculated for each subject and scores for the two groups were compared (table 5). There were significant differences in both day and night scores with children in the intervention group having fewer symptoms. There was no between group difference in the disability score.

We did not monitor how often families in the two groups used the oral steroids provided.

Discussion

Despite a widespread consensus about the treatment of acute childhood asthma,[15 17] the outcome – at least as reflected in the number of hospital re-admissions – is disappointing.[3 4] In this pragmatic, prospective, randomised control study we examined the impact of the introduction of a brief, structured, nurse-led asthma home management training programme administered during admission. The outcome was clear. In the children randomised to receive usual asthma treatment 25% were re-admitted during the study period (individual follow up 2–14 months). This was similar to the number of re-admissions in the group not randomised (table 3), to our own previous observations, and to published data.[3] In striking

Table 4 Parameter estimates for re-admission in the Cox proportional hazards model

Variable	*Estimate of coefficient*	*Estimated standard error*	*Hazard ratio**	*95% confidence interval*
One previous admission	1.3816	0.6363	3.98	(1.12 to 14.21)
Two or more previous admissions	2.1207	0.5572	8.34	(2.74 to 25.41)
Intervention	−0.9486	0.4236	0.39	(0.17 to 0.90)

*The ratio of the hazard function for children with the given feature compared with the hazard function for a baseline control group with no previous admission.

contrast, re-admissions fell significantly from 25% to 8% in the intervention group. This decrease in re-admissions was not accompanied by any subsequent increase in emergency room use nor, at least in the short term, by any increase in the reported attendance for urgent community asthma treatment immediately following discharge. The intervention group also showed significant reductions in day and night morbidity scores assessed using a morbidity questionnaire 3–4 weeks after discharge from hospital.

While the attending medical staff were fully aware of the study, it was designed not to interfere with their established clinical practice. For the intervention group the aim was to complement but not supplant or alter usual management. Consequently, the results in the intervention group are all the more striking when it is noted that differences in the medical management of the acute episode, in the length of stay, in the prescribed inhaled therapy at discharge, and in planned medical follow up were, indeed, minimal.

In this study we did not investigate behavioural or educational outcomes. Other studies have clearly shown that asthma education programmes can improve asthma knowledge and treatment compliance. Bernard-Bonnin *et al*[18] have pointed out that these outcomes are more directly related to the teaching intervention and are therefore likely to be less susceptible to confounding factors that might "dilute" the impact of teaching interventions on measures of morbidity. In using re-admission as the primary outcome we have, in effect, used a more rigorous test of the impact of our programme.

Like Mitchell *et al*,[4] we noted that the number of previous admissions was a significant risk factor for re-admission. We did not find that characteristics of the individual (age and sex) or severity of the condition (as reflected in oxygen saturation at admission, use of intravenous theophylline) influenced re-admission. In particular, there was no evidence that the use of intravenous theophylline was associated with a decreased risk of re-admission. However, there were very substantial differences in our practice where 8–10% of children received intravenous theophylline compared with 98% in Mitchell's study. The differences in average age between the studies probably reflect the fact that our study excluded children below two years.

The individualised asthma management plans developed for children under five were based on symptoms. In children over five years of age a peak flow meter was issued but the plans were developed in terms of both symptoms and peak flow and parents were given the option of using which ever they preferred. The success of a symptom based approach in this childhood population echoes the findings of Charlton *et al*.[15] One important feature of our teaching programme was to provide parents with a check list of prodromal features of acute asthma to compare with their own experience.[12] We think this encouraged them to use their experience of their child's attacks as the basis for the recognition and management of future episodes. Although the teaching programme was relatively brief, it embodied a number of elements that have been identified as "principles of behaviour change and health education" such as the use of multiple methods, individualisation, relevance, feedback, and reinforcement.[19]

There are a number of other important points which should be emphasised. Although Glasgow has a high rate of urban deprivation, confirmed in the children studied by deprivation scores based on post code (table 1),[15] the training programme was introduced in a health care system free at the point of access. Thus financial constraints were unlikely to limit or bias the population studied.

Most importantly, perhaps, the study was not restricted to children having their first asthma admission with the median number of previous admissions being two, thus reflecting children with more severe asthma. Mitchell *et al* also studied an educational programme in similar children admitted to hospital with asthma.[20] However, in contrast, they found subsequent hospital admissions were increased in the intervention group. Two important differences from that study should be highlighted. Our teaching programme was delivered during admission when parents may be particularly receptive. Clark *et al*[21] have also noted a significant reduction in both use of the emergency room and admissions to hospital with self-management training when comparison was restricted to a small group of children who had been admitted to hospital during the preceding year. Similarly, Osman *et al* found that hospital admission seemed to offer an opportunity to influence patient self-management behaviour and the later risk of re-admission in adult asthmatic patients.[22] Hospital admission may therefore be a key window of opportunity for maximising the impact of home management training programmes.

Another important difference from the study by Mitchell may be that we provided the parents with a short course of oral corticosteroids with instructions to start this if an exacerbation occurred, avoiding delay due either to a delay in consulting their family doctor or to reluctance of the doctor to start corticosteroids. We did not, however, monitor how frequently courses of oral steroids were started in the two groups.

It has been suggested that re-admissions within 72 hours of hospital admission might be an outcome indicator reflecting the quality of hospital asthma care. We found that re-admissions in both groups were very uncommon immediately after the index admission (fig 1). As a consequence, this outcome is not likely to be a useful index of the quality of care. Instead, we suggest that asthma re-admissions over a much longer time are a better outcome indicator. Avoiding any subsequent admission should then be a major health care goal in childhood asthma.

Because of limited resources, the study training programme was always delivered by one specialist nurse. While this immediately ensured consistency in implementation, it potentially raises questions about the generalisability of our findings. Notwithstanding, the study showed that substantial reductions in readmissions can be achieved; the challenge now is to realise these reductions in regular practice. The pragmatic randomised introduction has provided evidence to justify extending the programme to all asthmatic children aged over two years admitted to our hospital and has provided a benchmark against which to monitor our subsequent progress.

1 Strachan DP, Anderson HR. Trends in hospital admission rates for asthma in children. *BMJ* 1992;304:819–20.
2 Anderson HR. Increase in hospital admissions for childhood asthma: trends in referral, severity, and readmissions from 1970 to 1985 in a health region of the United Kingdom. *Thorax* 1989;44:614–9.
3 Senthilsevan A. Effect of readmissions on increasing hospital admissions for asthma in children. *Thorax* 1995;50:934–6.
4 Mitchell EA, Bland JM, Thomson JMD. Risk factors for readmission to hospital for asthma in childhood. *Thorax* 1994;49:33–6.
5 Mitchell EA, Cutler DR. Paediatric admissions to Auckland Hospital for asthma from 1970–1980. *N Z Med J* 1984; 97:67–70.
6 Thoresen CE, Kirmil-Gray K. Self-management psychology and the treatment of childhood asthma. *J Allergy Clin Immunol* 1983;72:596–606.
7 Rachelefsky GS. Review of asthma self-management programs. *J Allergy Clin Immunol* 1987;80:506–11.
8 Howland J, Bauchner H, Adair R. The impact of pediatric asthma education on morbidity. Assessing the evidence. *Chest* 1988;94:964–9.
9 Klingelhofer EL, Gershwin ME. Asthma self management programs: premises, not promises. *J Asthma* 1988;25: 89–101.
10 Bernard-Bonnin A-C, Stachenko S, Bonin D, Charette C, Rousseau E. Self-management teaching programs and morbidity of paediatric asthma: a meta-analysis. *J Allergy Clin Immunol* 1995;95:34–41.
11 Silverman M. Out of the mouths of babes and sucklings: lessons from early childhood asthma. *Thorax* 1993;48: 1200–4.
12 Beer S, Laver J, Karpuch J, Chabut S, Aladjem M. Prodromal features of asthma. *Arch Dis Child* 1987;62:345–8.
13 D'Souza W, Crane J, Burgess C, Te Karu H, Fox C, Harper M, *et al.* Community-based asthma care: trial of a "credit card" asthma self-management plan. *Eur Respir J* 1994;7: 1260–5.
14 Usherwood TP, Scrimgeour A, Barber JH. Questionnaire to measure perceived symptoms and disability in asthma. *Arch Dis Child* 1990;65:779–81.
15 Carstairs V, Morris R. Deprivation: explaining differences in mortality between Scotland and England and Wales. *BMJ* 1989;299:886–9.
16 National Heart Lung and Blood Institute. International consensus report on diagnosis and treatment of asthma. Bethesda, Maryland: Department of Health and Human Services, 1992.
17 International Paediatric Consensus Group. Asthma: a follow-up statement from an international paediatric consensus group. *Arch Dis Child* 1992;67:240–8.
18 Charlton I, Charlton G, Broomfield J, Mullee MA. Evaluation of peak flow and symptoms on self management plans for control of asthma in general practice. *BMJ* 1990; 301:1355–9.
19 Green LW, Frankish CJ. Theories and principles of health education applied to asthma. *Chest* 1994;106:219–30S.
20 Mitchell EA, Ferguson V, Norwood M. Asthma education by community child health nurses. *Arch Dis Child* 1986; 61:1184–9.
21 Clark NM, Feldman CH, Evans D, Levison MJ, Wasilewski Y, Mellins RB. The impact of health education on frequency and cost of health care use by low income children with asthma. *J Allergy Clin Immunol* 1986;78:108–15.
22 Osman LM, Friend JAR, Legge JS, Douglas JG. Successful avoidance of hospital re-admission in acute asthma. *Eur Respir J* 1994;7:13s.

Clinical question:

Are the results of this single preventive or therapeutic trial valid?

Was the assignment of patients to treatments randomised?
Was the randomisation list concealed?

Were all patients who entered the trial accounted for at its conclusion?
Were they analysed in the groups to which they were randomised?

Were patients and clinicians kept 'blind' to which treatment was being received?

Aside from the experimental treatment, were the groups treated equally?

Were the groups similar at the start of the trial?

Are the valid results of this randomised trial important?

SAMPLE CALCULATIONS (*see* pp 134–40 of *Evidence-based Medicine*)

Occurrence of diabetic neuropathy		**Relative risk reduction (RRR)**	**Absolute risk reduction (ARR)**	**Number needed to treat (NNT)**
Usual insulin control event rate (CER)	Intensive insulin experimental event rate (EER)	$\frac{\text{CER} - \text{EER}}{\text{CER}}$	CER – EER	1 / ARR
9.6%	2.8%	$\frac{9.6\% - 2.8\%}{9.6\%}$ = 71%	9.6% – 2.8% = 6.8%	1 / 6.8% = 15 pts

95% confidence interval (CI) on an NNT = 1 / (limits on the CI of its ARR) =

$$+/-1.96\sqrt{\frac{\text{CER}\times(1-\text{CER})}{\#\text{ of control pts}}+\frac{\text{EER}\times(1-\text{EER})}{\#\text{ of exper. pts}}} = +/-1.96\sqrt{\frac{0.096\times 0.904}{730}+\frac{0.028\times 0.972}{711}} = \pm 2.4\%$$

YOUR CALCULATIONS

		Relative risk reduction (RRR)	**Absolute risk reduction (ARR)**	**Number needed to treat (NNT)**
CER	EER	$\frac{\text{CER} - \text{EER}}{\text{CER}}$	CER – EER	1 / ARR

Can you apply this valid, important evidence about a treatment in caring for your patient?

Do these results apply to your patient?

Is your patient so different from those in the trial that its results can't help you?

How great would the potential benefit of therapy actually be for your individual patient?

Method I: **f**	(a) Risk of the outcome in your patient without R, relative to patients in the trial, expressed as a decimal:_____ (b) NNT/f = ___/___ = (c) NNT for patients like yours
Method II: **1 / (PEER × RRR)**	(a) Your patient's expected event rate if they received the control treatment: PEER:______ (b) 1 / (PEER × RRR) = 1 /______ = _______ (c) NNT for patients like yours
Method III: **1 / PEER – (PEER × Relative risk)**	(a) Your patient's expected event rate if they received the control treatment: PEER:______ (b) Relative risk – EER/CER =______ (c) 1 / PEER – (PEER × Relative risk) =______ (d) NNT for patients like yours

Are your patient's values and preferences satisfied by the regimen and its consequences?

Does your patient and you have a clear assessment of their values and preferences?

Are they met by this regimen and its consequences?

Additional notes

COMPLETED THERAPY WORKSHEET: 1 of 2

Clinical question: In children with asthma, does a nurse-led asthma programme (compared to no programme) lead to reduced readmission rates?

Are the results of this single preventive or therapeutic trial valid?

Was the assignment of patients to treatments randomised? Was the randomisation list concealed?	**Yes.** **Yes, performed before the study.**
Were all patients who entered the trial accounted for at its conclusion?	**Yes, for readmission (not for morbidity questionnaire). Some children followed for 2 mths instead of 14 mths, but survival curve (Fig 1) shows intervention still significant.**
Were they analysed in the groups to which they were randomised?	**Yes.**
Were patients and clinicians kept 'blind' to which treatment was being received?	**Uncertain. Staff responsible for readmission should have been blind, but the parents were not.**
Aside from the experimental treatment, were the groups treated equally?	**No. Intervention group was given oral steroids to start at home.**
Were the groups similar at the start of the trial?	**No. Median age was higher in intervention group (Table 1). However, data stratified by age and analysed by Cox's proportional hazard analysis and results still significant.**

Are the valid results of this randomised trial important?

YOUR CALCULATIONS

		Relative risk reduction (RRR)	Absolute risk reduction (ARR)	Number needed to treat (NNT)
CER	EER	$\frac{CER - EER}{CER}$	CER – EER	1 / ARR
24.8%	8.3%	67%	16.5%	6

95% confidence interval (CI) on a NNT = 1 / (limits on CI of its ARR)

$$+/-1.96\sqrt{\frac{CER \times (1-CER)}{\text{\# of control pts}} + \frac{EER \times (1-EER)}{\text{\# of exper. pts}}} = +/-1.96\sqrt{\frac{0.248 \times 0.752}{105} + \frac{0.083 \times 0.917}{96}}$$

= 4 to 16 (does not include 0 so is statistically significant)

Can you apply this valid, important evidence about a treatment in caring for your patient?

Do these results apply to your patient?

Is your patient so different from those in the trial that its results can't help you?	**No. Patients similar, but is your nurse trainer similar?**

How great would the potential benefit of therapy actually be for your individual patient?

Method I: **f** **your readmission rate is 18%**	(a) Risk of the outcome in your patient, relative to patients in the trial, expressed as a decimal: 0.18 / 0.248 = 0.73 (b) NNT/f = 6 / 0.73 = 8 (c) NNT for patients like yours 8
Method II: **1 / (PEER × RRR)**	(a) Your patient's expected event rate if they received the control treatment: PEER: 18% (b) 1 / (PEER × RRR) = 1 / (0.18 × 0.67) = 8 (c) NNT for patients like yours 8
Method III: **1 / PEER – (PEER × relative risk)**	(a) PEER = 18% (b) Relative risk – EER/CER = 0.33 (c) 1 / PEER – (PEER × RR) = 1/0.12 = 8 (d) NNT for patients like yours 8

Are your patient's values and preferences satisfied by the regimen and its consequences?

Does your patient and you have a clear assessment of their values and preferences?	**Appropriateness of home training needs to be assessed in each patient.**
Are they met by this regimen and its consequences?	**Appropriateness of home training needs to be assessed in each patient.**

Additional notes

1. Method 3 for finding NNT : Look at reciprocal of absolute risk difference (ARR).
   Relative risk (RR) = EER/CER = 8.3/24.8 = 33%. If your CER is 18% or 0.18, then with intervention, your EER is 0.33 × 0.18 = 0.059 or 6%
   ARR = 18% – 6% = 12%; NNT = 1/0.12 = 8
2. From patient point of view, intervention seems good, but not from GP point of view as increased GP attendance in intervention group.
3. Readmission rate in your unit is low anyway and you may decide to use scarce resources in other ways.
4. The intervention was a package and it is not possible to say which element of the package produced the effect.

ASTHMA – NURSE-LED HOME MANAGEMENT TRAINING PROGRAMME REDUCED READMISSION FOR ASTHMA

Appraised by O Duperrex and R Gilbert: 12 February 1999
Expiry date: February 2000.

Clinical Bottom Line

In children of 2 or more years hospitalised for asthma, readmission rate can be reduced by a nurse-led package of education and support (NNT = 6 for a baseline risk of 25%).

Citation

Madge P, McColl J and Paton J (1997) Impact of a nurse-led home management training programme in children admitted to hospital with acute asthma: a randomised controlled study. *Thorax* **52**(3): 223–8.

Clinical Question

In children hospitalised for asthma, can a nurse-led home asthma management programme reduce readmission for asthma?

Search Terms

'asthma' and 'child' and 'patient-readmission' and 'randomised-controlled-trial'.

The Study

1 Randomised controlled trial with adequate concealment of randomisation, objective assessment of the main outcome and an intention-to-treat analysis.
2 Study patients were children aged 2 or more years who were randomised on admission for asthma.
3 Control group (N = 105) received 'usual care' and were not aware of the study.
4 Experimental group (N = 96) received on average 45 minutes education with a single asthma-nurse specialist, written information and advice, telephone support after discharge and a course of oral steroids to start at home when required.

The Evidence:

Outcome	Time to Outcome	EER	CER	RRR	ARR	NNT
Hospital readmission for asthma	2–14 months	0.083	0.248	67%	0.165	6
95% confidence intervals				29–84%	0.07–0.26	4–16

Comments

1 The intervention group also had a significant reduction in symptoms 3–4 weeks after discharge and no evidence of an increase in attendance at A&E or the GP.
2 Which element of the package produced the effect: education, written information, telephone support or the provision of a course of oral corticosteroids for parents to start when symptoms recurred?
3 Generalisation of findings reflecting intervention by one nurse should be made with caution.

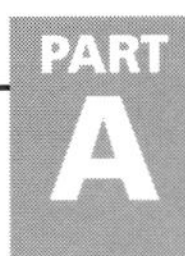

Critical appraisal of a clinical article about therapy

EBCH SESSION

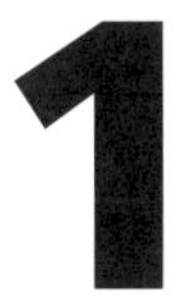

SECTION 2

Therapy and introduction to CATS

Section 2: Postal reminders for vaccination uptake

You are a community paediatrician and are concerned that your immunisation rate has fallen to 82%.

One of the health visitors asks if changing the computerised reminder card might improve rates. Your present reminder card is thought to be too impersonal.

You decide to undertake a search to find out if there are any studies on uptake rates. You formulate the question, in my community, would modification of the postal reminder card based on a health belief model improve the immunisation uptake?

What, if any, changes do you decide to make? How will you make a case for the additional resources required to make any changes to the vaccination reminder system?

Search strategy for postal reminders for vaccination uptake

Type in:
1 measles vaccination in TI,AB,Mesh
2 explode "Measles-Vaccine" / all subheadings
3 measles-vaccine in TI,AB,Mesh
4 #1 cr #2 #3
5 postal reminder in TI,AB,Mesh
6 uptake in TI,AB,Mesh
7 #4 and #5 and #6

Using this strategy you find the article by Hawe *et al.* (*Arch Dis Child* 1998; **79:** 136–40)

Read the article and decide:
1 Is the evidence from this randomised trial valid?
2 If valid, is this evidence important?
3 If valid and important, can you apply this evidence in caring for your patient?

If you want to read some strategies for answering these sorts of questions, you could have a look at pp 91–6, 133–41 and 166–72 in *Evidence-based Medicine*.

PART B

How to use the CATMaker (optional)

If a CATMaker is provided with this package you will be shown how to use it to generate and save your own one page 'critically appraised topic' (CAT) from an article about therapy. The advantages of the CATMaker include its ability to calculate for you the clinically useful measures of the effects of therapy and their confidence intervals, and to save your critical appraisal for printing, sharing and storage.

Randomised controlled trial of the use of a modified postal reminder card on the uptake of measles vaccination

P Hawe, N McKenzie, R Scurry

Abstract

***Objective*—To determine whether rewording postal reminder cards according to the "health belief model", a theory about preventive health behaviour, would help to improve measles vaccination rates.**

***Design*—A randomised controlled trial, with blind assessment of outcome status. Parents of children due for their first measles vaccination were randomised to one of two groups, one receiving the health belief model reminder card, the other receiving the usual, neutrally worded card. The proportion of children subsequently vaccinated in each group over a five week period was ascertained from clinical (provider based) records.**

***Setting*—A local government operated public vaccination clinic.**

***Participants*—Parents of 259 children due for measles vaccination.**

***Main results*—The proportion of children vaccinated in the health belief model card group was 79% compared with 67% of those sent the usual card (95% CI, 2% to 23%), a modest but important improvement.**

***Conclusion*—This study illustrates how the effectiveness of a minimal and widely practised intervention to promote vaccination compliance can be improved with negligible additional effort.**

(*Arch Dis Child* 1998;79:136–140)

Keywords: measles vaccination; postal reminders; randomised controlled trial; health promotion

Studies of postal reminder systems for vaccination have appeared in the literature since the early 1960s,[1] and the impact of computer assisted registries has been evaluated in the UK,[2] Canada,[3] and New Zealand.[4] Recently, a national computer based registry and postal reminder system has been established in Australia, as part of a renewed national strategy to improve childhood vaccination rates.[5] Increasingly, however, the call for evidence based practice has led to a re-examination of many widespread practices in both health care and public health. In childhood vaccination, a systematic review of parent level interventions (such as reminder systems) by Tannenbaum and his colleagues in 1994 concluded that there was insufficient evidence to recommend that they be routine practice for measles/mumps/rubella vaccination or diphtheria/pertussis/tetanus vaccination.[6] This was because of the relatively weak methods used in most studies up until that time and insufficient accumulation of evidence from the few studies that were rated as moderate or strong. However, a most striking feature of previous evaluations of childhood vaccination reminders is the extent to which they have ignored theory and research in health behaviour. Researchers have not given much thought to the way that messages should be framed. Indeed, very few studies have reported the content of the messages, with a notable exception being the study by Stehr-Green *et al* pertaining to telephone reminders.[7] We would argue that by failing to appraise critically the content of the reminders along with the quality of the study design, systematic reviews in vaccination have given us only a partial view of the potential of particular interventions. The design of preventive interventions is not "common sense". Indeed, there is a possibility that so-called motivational mailings about vaccination, designed in ignorance of theories about health behaviour,[8] might in fact be counter productive.[9] One popular health behaviour theory is the "health belief model". It states that people will be more likely to undertake a health behaviour if they feel that: (1) the disease in question is severe, (2) they are susceptible to it, and (3) the action that is recommended will have benefits that will outweigh any associated costs.[10] The health belief model was developed in the early 1950s by social psychologists in the US Public Health Service attempting to explain the widespread failure of people to participate in preventive health programmes, particularly *x* ray screening programmes in tuberculosis control.[11] Extensively researched since that time, its predictive validity in relation to a wide range of health behaviours has been the subject of review[12] and meta analysis.[13] High quality intervention studies with the health belief model have been relatively few.[11] Although there is some limited evidence that vaccination reminders based on the health belief model could increase adult vaccination rates,[14] no researchers appear to have tested the usefulness of the model in relation to any of the routine childhood vaccinations. We set out to determine whether postal reminders reworded according to the health belief model could improve vaccination rates for measles.

Methods

The study was conducted with a municipal council within the provincial city of Ballarat (regional population, 70 000). The council had

Department of Public Health and Community Medicine (A27), University of Sydney, NSW 2006, Australia
P Hawe

Health Department, City of Ballarat
N McKenzie

Health Department, City of Ballarat
R Scurry

Correspondence to:
Dr Hawe.

Accepted 4 February 1998

Ballarat City Council

Dear Mrs QUINN,

MEASLES is still a problem in Ballarat, particularly for children under the age of 2 years. Some children suffer severe complications.

The children who are most likely to catch measles are those who have not been immunised. Immunisation is very effective. There is almost no chance of side effects. Clinics are held at the Lower Civic Hall in Mair Street from 2 - 3.40 pm EVERY SECOND WEDNESDAY. Immunisations are given by a doctor. Of course, immunisation is free!

The next clinic is on Wednesday 14th December. If GEORGIA is not yet immunised against measles, you should bring her along.

Regards,
Bob Scurry
HEALTH DEPARTMENT
Enquiries: ph 313 277

Figure 1 Health belief model card.

CITY OF BALLARAT

Dear Parent, (as addressed)

Council records indicate that Georgia
is due/overdue for the following vaccination:

TRIPLE ANTIGEN	1ST	2ND	3RD	CDT
POLIOMYELITIS	1ST	2ND	3RD	4TH
MEASLES/MUMPS		TRIPLE ANTIGEN BOOSTER		

Please present your child with this card for vaccination at the Lower Civic Hall at 2 pm on 14 December
If unable to attend or wish to change the appointment date, or you do not wish to continue, continuing elswhere, or changing address, please contact the HEALTH DEPARTMENT, TOWN HALL, STURT STREET, BALLARAT. PHONE: 31 3277

Figure 2 Usual vaccination reminder card sent by the council.

an existing computerised reminder system. The content and main features of the health belief model card were derived from the literature.[12-14] We decided that the use of a no intervention control group, rather than a usual intervention control group, might yield a greater margin of difference compared with the experimental health belief model intervention, but that this would be an undesirable, artificial test scenario, given that postal reminder cards systems were widespread. Thus, the question being asked in our trial was not: "Shall we do 'X' or shall we do nothing?" but rather: "What can we add to existing practice to improve health outcomes?" A series of four focus groups was conducted to pretest the health belief model card. These were held with parents from the target group considered to be hardest to reach with written messages—that is, people with low socioeconomic status, and minimal education. Parents were recruited for the focus groups by social and welfare workers in the surrounding municipalities—that is, areas outside the one within which the trial was to be conducted. As a result of these groups, the health belief model card was altered in a number of ways. Words such as "susceptible" were dropped because of parents' limited understanding. The title of the person who sends the card (the Chief Health Surveyor) was also dropped because it was viewed as intimidating. The card was signed from the "Health Department" instead. The final card was addressed specifically to the parent ("Dear Mrs Quinn" instead of "Dear Parent") and the child was referred to by name. The final format and wording of the health belief model card is illustrated in fig 1. The usual neutrally worded card sent by the council clinic appears in fig 2.

The study population comprised the parents of children born consecutively between 24 August 1987 and 28 February 1988, who were due for measles vaccination—that is, the children who reached 15 months of age during the study period (the recommended age for vaccination in Australia has since been reduced to 12 months of age). Children were identified from the municipal council lists, which are based on birth notifications supplied by local hospitals. The lists are thought to cover at least 98% of children in this age group in the municipality.[15] The birth dates listed above encompassed 300 children, although it was agreed in advance that a single interim analysis would be conducted when approximately 262 children had been recruited into the study, and the trial stopped if a difference was significant at the 5% level. This sample size calculation was based on an expectation of the difference between the "health belief model" card and the usual card being in the order of 15%, drawing on the results of a pilot study of 60 children and estimating the vaccination rate in the control group to be 70% (significance level of 5% and power of 80%).[16] Parents of the 300 children due to receive measles vaccination reminders were allocated randomly into two groups, one to receive the usual card and one to receive the health belief model card. After randomisation and before cards were sent, the council was notified of the death of one child and two further children were vaccinated early by private medical practitioners. These three children were excluded from the analysis. After cards were sent to the remaining children, 10 cards were returned because the addresses were incorrect, or the family had moved. Nine cards were not sent because of administrative error. Cards were sent in batches according to when a child became due for vaccination. A vaccination clinic was held one week after cards were sent. The next clinic was two weeks later. Parents who did not have their children vaccinated at either of these first two clinics were sent a second reminder card, which was the same type as the first card they had been sent. Another clinic was held a week after the second card had been sent. After this time the final proportion of children who had been vaccinated in both groups was determined. A child was coded as "vaccination having been received" if the parent presented to any of the three clinics held after the first reminder card had been sent. We were also advised, by usual reciprocal arrangement with neighbouring councils, if any of the parents in our study group had their child vaccinated by a neighbouring council. We were also aware if a child had been vaccinated during this period by a private medical practitioner either because: (1) a parent volunteered this information upon receipt of our second reminder (and the medical practitioner could be named and the report verified); or (2) because the medical practitioner had advised us directly, as part of the usual arrangement

Table 1 Sociodemograhic characteristics of study groups

	HBM card (n = 90)	Usual card (n = 83)	Difference (95% CI)	p value
Mean number of children in family	2.1	2.3	−0.2 (−0.12, 0.55)	0.21
Mean number of children ≤ 5 years	1.6	1.8	−0.2 (−0.05, 0.32)	0.14
Mean mother's age	29.8	30.0	−0.2 (−1.28, 1.8)	0.74
Mean number of years mother at high school	4.9	4.6	0.3 (−0.6, 0.03)	0.072
Mother born in Australia	96%	92%	4% (−3, 11)	0.22
Mean father's age	33.1	32.2	0.9 (−2.7, 0.97)	0.35
Mean number of years father at high school	4.6	4.5	0.0 (−0.45, 0.33)	0.77
Father born in Australia	91%	90%	1% (−8, 11)	0.78
Single parent family	12%	5%	7% (−1, 15)	0.08
Dependent on pension/benefit	13%	9%	4% (−6, 13)	0.45

HBM, health belief model.

regarding distribution of vaccines by the council to doctors and agreement by doctors to report who they vaccinate to the council. The administrative assistant recording the vaccinations was not aware of what type of card a parent had received. At the conclusion of the trial, all parents in the trial sample were sent a self administered questionnaire to determine their sociodemographic characteristics. This step was taken at the end of the study rather than at the beginning to avoid the possibility of sensitising parents about the vaccination clinic and the Health Department before the postal trial was conducted. It was explained that the purpose of the questionnaire was to find out parents' views about the quality of the vaccination clinics and mode of transport used to get to clinics. This generated useful information secondary to the study purpose. The sociodemographic questionnaire included a number of sensitive questions (household composition and dependency on social security payments) and, as such, the decision was taken that it should be completed and returned anonymously, in order to maximise response rates. The only identifying information on the questionnaire was a symbol that identified the group membership of the respondent. This decision meant that personally identifying sociodemographic information could not be linked to vaccination rates in the subsequent analysis. Ethics approval for the study was received from the University of Melbourne. The analysis was conducted when 259 children had been recruited into the study, 124 into the health belief model card group and 135 into the usual card group. This was just short of the intended number because of failure to move the cut off point to compensate for the three excluded children (an error). The analysis was conducted using the principle of intention to treat—all eligible subjects were included in the analysis. The 10 children whose cards were returned because the parents had moved or the cards were not correctly addressed were considered "late ineligibles"[17] and were included in the analysis. The nine children whose cards were not sent because of administrative error were ruled eligible and were included in the analysis. Two sample t tests and χ^2 analyses were conducted using the Minitab statistical package. The 95% confidence intervals to test the differences between the proportions were calculated using the formula supplied by Bland.[18]

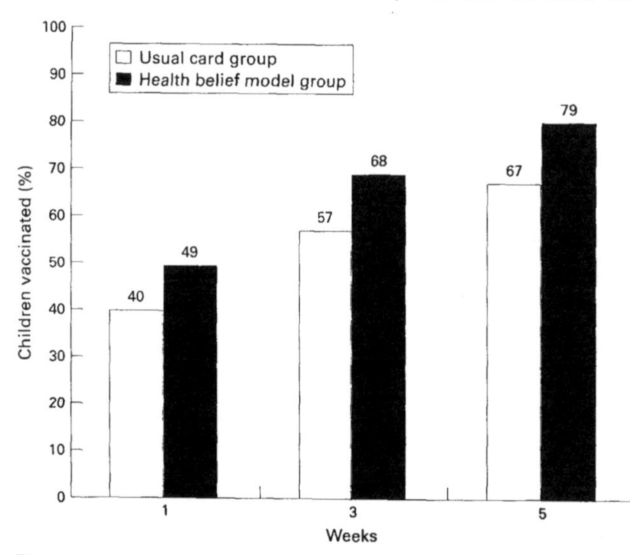

Figure 3 Percentage of children vaccinated in the five weeks following a postal reminder prompt.

Results

The sociodemographic characteristics of the two groups in the study are illustrated in table 1. One hundred and seventy three questionnaires (67%) were returned after two attempts. Seventy one per cent of questionnaires were returned from the health belief model card group and 62% of questionnaires were returned from the usual card group. Apparent differences between the groups in table 1 (which are not significant) might possibly reflect a difference in those who returned the questionnaire rather than real differences between the groups, although the direction of bias, if any exists, is against the health belief model group. No additional data sources were available to determine whether the sociodemographic characteristics of those parents who returned the questionnaire differed from those who did not. The sample was almost entirely Australian born, a result that would be expected for a large country town in Australia, but would be unusual for large metropolitan areas. Other countries of birth represented in the sample include the UK, the Netherlands, Yugoslavia, Hong Kong, and Vietnam.

In the assessment of outcome, the 10 children who were lost to follow up (five in the health belief model group and five in the usual card group), for whom vaccination status was not known, appeared in the denominator and were counted as unvaccinated in the numerator (that is, the worse case scenario was assumed). The nine children whose cards were not sent were included in the denominator, and were included in the numerator according to their vaccination status. Three children in the health belief model group did not receive cards, one of whom was vaccinated, and six children in the usual card group did not receive cards, one of whom was vaccinated. The effectiveness of the health belief model card compared to the usual card is presented in fig 3. At the conclusion of the study, 79% (98 children) of the "health belief model" card group were vaccinated compared with 67% (90 children) of the usual card group. This is a difference of 12%, which is significant (95% CI, 2% to 23%; $\chi^2 = 4.967$; df = 1; p = 0.026). The significance of the difference between the groups was not sensitive to alternative handling of the 19 children who did not receive reminder cards. That is, the results remain significant with the 10 children with incorrect addresses removed (n = 249; $\chi^2 = 5.784$; df = 1; p = 0.016), or with all 19 removed from the analysis (n = 240; $\chi^2 = 4.824$; df = 1; p = 0.028).

Discussion

In this study, a 12% improvement in vaccination rate was seen when a health belief model vaccination reminder card was used instead of the usual card sent by the council. However, it should be noted that the additional contribution of wording the card personally to the parent and signing it personally by a council officer might have enhanced the effect. That is, the effect size of the health belief model seen here is confounded by the additional effort made to personalise the card. Also, in the health belief model group, parents were given slightly more information about the location of the vaccination clinic, although the effect of this is considered to be negligible, given that all parents had visited the clinic up to 12 months before to receive the triple antigen vaccine. We took the view that the purpose of the trial was to maximise the effect of a postal reminder card, not to test the health belief model in a pure sense, and hence factors that added to the card's appeal were included. Although a significant 12% improvement was seen with the health belief model card, because the trial was stopped when the number of participants reached 259, the estimate of effect was less precise. A larger sample size would have narrowed the confidence intervals around the estimate of effect. The council was not keen to continue the trial once a clear effect had been shown for two reasons. The first was the desire to put the new card (if successful) into place, the second was to cut short the disruption caused by the additional workload of data collection. Nine cards were not sent in this trial because of administrative error. Incorrect or out of date addresses also thwarted the potential of the strategy being tested. Hence, the size of the effect observed here was diluted, and could have been higher. Registries will vary in the extent to which lists are up to date and in the degree of administrative attention they receive for upkeep of reminder systems. Hence, the effect of the card will vary in different settings. Stehr-Green and colleagues[7] noted a similar problem in their randomised trial of a telephone computer generated reminder for childhood vaccinations. One fifth of their inner city sample could not be reached by telephone. The primary analysis by intention to treat showed a slight effect of only marginal significance, but an analysis among the subgroup who were reached by the telephone call showed a significant difference of 11% between the experimental and the (no intervention) control groups. A similar reinvestigation in our study of those who were known to have received cards (that is, excluding 19 children) adjusts the vaccination level in the experimental group from 79% to 84% and the corresponding levels in the control group from 67% to 72%. However, it should be emphasised that such analyses effectively remove the "real life" conditions to which results of trials actually should be generalised and, as such, these types of analyses are generally discouraged.[19]

The differential response rate to the follow up questionnaire is difficult to interpret. We can only speculate that the parents receiving the health belief model card noticed and appreciated the card, were more likely to act upon it, and subsequently took more interest in returning a questionnaire about their opinion on council run services. The groups did not differ in the types of comments made about clinic services—that is, whether their remarks were positive or negative. The study population for this trial was predominantly Australian born. Although other investigators have shown that the health belief model is also a useful framework for analysing childhood vaccination behaviour in cross cultural contexts,[20] we believe that the results here cannot be extrapolated to different ethnic groups. Appropriate formative research would be required to develop tailor written vaccination messages in other languages. In our study, 21% of the parents who received the health belief model card did not respond to the invitation to vaccinate their child in the following few weeks. Clearly, a range of factors affect vaccination compliance, only some of which can be addressed simply by increasing the sophistication of our written messages about vaccination importance. However, it is significant that the study has shown that with negligible additional effort, the effectiveness of a widely established strategy to promote vaccination compliance can be improved. Other investigators have also shown that the health belief model might be used to provide greater improvements in health outcomes in preventive medicine,[13] although it should be noted that the apparent margin of benefit is likely to vary according to what the control group receives and according to situational conditions. For example, with regard to influenza vaccination reminders to parents of children with asthma, Szilagyi *et al* found a very large margin of difference conferred by the health belief model, in that 30% of children whose parents received a health belief model card were vaccinated compared with just 7% in a no intervention control group.[21] Compared with many other countries, high routine childhood vaccination levels are already being achieved in the UK (although population pockets with lower vaccination rates might remain).[22] In such circumstances, the degree of benefit that could be conferred by rewording vaccination postal reminders according to the health belief model is uncertain. However, complacency about vaccination levels should be avoided. Because universal vaccination is the goal, all possibilities for improvements on the margin, with minimal additional cost, are worthy of consideration.

This study was carried out with assistance from a National Health and Medical Research Council Public Health Research Fellowship granted to the first author and a Measles Immunisation Grant from the Victorian Department of Health.

1 Galloway T. Management of vaccination and immunisation procedures by electronic computer. *Med Officer* 1963;**109**:232–3.
2 Bussey AL, Harris AS. Computers and the effectiveness of the measles vaccination campaign in England and Wales. *Commun Med* 1979;**1**:29–35.
3 Loeser H, Zvagulis I, Hercz L, Pless B. The organisation and evaluation of a computer assisted centralised immunisation registry. *Am J Public Health* 1983:**74**:1298–300.
4 Reid JS, Graham-Smith HJ. Childhood immunisations: a recall system is worthwhile. *NZ Med J* 1984;**97**:688–9.
5 National Health and Medical Research Council. *National immunisation strategy.* Canberra: Australian Government Publishing Service, 1993.
6 Tannenbaum TN, Gyrokos T, Abrahamowicz M, *et al.* Immunisation delivery methods: practice recommendations. *Can J Public Health* 1994;**1**(suppl):S37–40.
7 Stehr-Green PA, Dini EF, Lindegren ML, Patriarca PA. Evaluation of telephone computer-generated reminders to improve immunisation coverage at inner city clinics. *Public Health Rep* 1993;**108**:426–30.
8 Byrne EB, Schaeffer W, Dini EF, Case GE. Infant immunisation surveillance: cost vs effect. *J Am Med Assoc* 1979;**212**:770–3.
9 Job RFS. Effective and ineffective use of fear in health promotion campaigns. *Am J Public Health* 1988;**78**:163–7.
10 Becker M, ed. The health belief model and personal health behaviour. *Health Educ Monogr* 1974;**2**:324–508.
11 Rosenstock IM. The health belief model: explaining behaviour through expectancies. In: Glanz K, Lewis FM, Rimer BK, eds. *Health behaviour and health education. Theory, research and practice.* San Francisco: Jossey Bass, 1990:39–62.
12 Janz NK, Becker MH. The health belief model. A decade later. *Health Educ Q* 1984;**11**:1–47.
13 Harrison JA, Mullen PD, Green LW. A meta-analysis of studies of the health belief model with adults. *Health Educ Res* 1992;**7**:107–16.
14 Larson EB, Bergman J, Heidrich F, Alvin BL, Schneeweiss R. Do postcards improve influenza vaccination compliance? *Med Care* 1982;**20**:639–48.
15 Thompson S. Programme management: immunisation in Victoria. Address to the 3rd National Immunisation Conference. Public Health Association of Australia. Melbourne, April 1993.
16 Casagrande T, Pike MC, Smith PG. The power function of the exact test for comparing binomial distributions. *Applied statistics* 1978;**27**:176–80.
17 Pocock SJ. *Clinical trials. A practical approach.* New York: John Wiley and Sons, 1985.
18 Bland M. *An introduction to medical statistics.* Oxford: Oxford Medical Publications, 1991.
19 Newell DJ. Intention to treat analysis: implications for quantitative and qualitative research. *Int J Epidemiol* 1992; **21**:837–41.
20 Eng E, Naimoli J, Naimoli G, Parker KA, Lowenthal N. The acceptability of childhood immunization to Togolese mothers: a sociobehavioural perspective. *Health Educ Q* 1991;**18**:97–110.
21 Szilagyi PG, Rodewald LE, Savageau J, Yoos L, Doane C. Improving influenza vaccination rates in children with asthma: a test of a computerised reminder system and an analysis of factors predicting vaccination compliance. *Pediatrics* 1992;**90**:871–5.
22 Reading R, Colver A, Openshaw S, Jarvis S. Do interventions that improve immunisation uptake also reduce inequalities in uptake? *BMJ* 1994;**308**:1142–4.

Clinical question:

Are the results of this single preventive or therapeutic trial valid?

Was the assignment of patients to treatments randomised?
Was the randomisation list concealed?

Were all patients who entered the trial accounted for at its conclusion?
Were they analysed in the groups to which they were randomised?

Were patients and clinicians kept 'blind' to which treatment was being received?

Aside from the experimental treatment, were the groups treated equally?

Were the groups similar at the start of the trial?

Are the valid results of this randomised trial important?

SAMPLE CALCULATIONS (*see* pp 134–40 of *Evidence-based Medicine*)

Occurrence of diabetic neuropathy		**Relative risk reduction (RRR)**	**Absolute risk reduction (ARR)**	**Number needed to treat (NNT)**
Usual insulin control event rate (CER)	Intensive insulin experimental event rate (EER)	$\frac{CER - EER}{CER}$	CER – EER	1 / ARR
9.6%	2.8%	$\frac{9.6\% - 2.8\%}{9.6\%}$ = 71%	9.6% – 2.8% = 6.8%	1 / 6.8% = 15 pts

95% confidence interval (CI) on an NNT = 1 / (limits on the CI of its ARR) =

$$+/-1.96\sqrt{\frac{CER \times (1-CER)}{\text{\# of control pts}} + \frac{EER \times (1-EER)}{\text{\# of exper. pts}}} = +/-1.96\sqrt{\frac{0.096 \times 0.904}{730} + \frac{0.028 \times 0.972}{711}} = \pm 2.4\%$$

YOUR CALCULATIONS

		Relative risk reduction (RRR)	**Absolute risk reduction (ARR)**	**Number needed to treat (NNT)**
CER	EER	$\frac{CER - EER}{CER}$	CER – EER	1 / ARR

Can you apply this valid, important evidence about a treatment in caring for your patient?

Do these results apply to your patient?

Is your patient so different from those in the trial that its results can't help you?

How great would the potential benefit of therapy actually be for your individual patient?

Method I: **f**	(a) Risk of the outcome in your patient, relative to patients in the trial, expressed as a decimal:_____ (b) NNT/f = ___/___ = (c) NNT for patients like yours
Method II: **1 / (PEER × RRR)**	(a) Your patient's expected event rate if they received the control treatment: PEER:______ (b) 1 / (PEER × RRR) = 1/______ = _______ (c) NNT for patients like yours
Method III: **1 / PEER – (PEER × Relative risk)**	(a) Your patient's expected event rate if they received the control treatment: PEER:______ (b) Relative risk – EER/CER =______ (c) 1 / PEER – (PEER × Relative risk) =______ (d) NNT for patients like yours

Are your patient's values and preferences satisfied by the regimen and its consequences?

Does your patient and you have a clear assessment of their values and preferences?

Are they met by this regimen and its consequences?

Additional notes

Clinical question:	In my community, would modification of the postal reminder card based on a health belief model, improve the immunisation uptake?

Are the results of this single preventive or therapeutic trial valid?

Was the assignment of patients to treatments randomised?	**Yes.**
Was the randomisation list concealed?	**Not stated.**
Were all patients who entered the trial accounted for at its conclusion?	**Yes.**
Were they analysed in the groups to which they were randomised?	**Yes.**
Were patients and clinicians kept 'blind' to which treatment was being received?	**No. Patients aware of reminder card they were sent (but not that it was a study). Clinic clerk unaware, ie. blind to treatment (so outcome measured objectively).**
Aside from the experimental treatment, were the groups treated equally?	**No, experimental group given an open appointment, whereas control group given fixed times.**
Were the groups similar at the start of the trial?	**Don't know, Table 1 is not informative.**

Are the valid results of this randomised trial important?

YOUR CALCULATIONS: Look at adverse outcome (i.e. risk of not being immunised)

		Relative risk reduction (RRR)	**Absolute risk reduction (ARR)**	**Number needed to treat (NNT)**
CER	EER	$\frac{\text{CER} - \text{EER}}{\text{CER}}$	CER – EER	1 / ARR
33%	21%	36%	12%	8

95% confidence interval (CI) on a NNT = 1 / (limits on CI of its ARR)

$$+/-1.96\sqrt{\frac{\text{CER}\times(1-\text{CER})}{\text{\# of control pts}}+\frac{\text{EER}\times(1-\text{EER})}{\text{\# of exper. pts}}} = +/-1.96\sqrt{\frac{0.33\times0.67}{135}+\frac{0.21\times0.79}{124}}$$

= 4 to 63 (does not include 0 so is statistically significant)

Can you apply this valid, important evidence about a treatment in caring for your patient?

Do these results apply to your patient?

Is your patient so different from those in the trial that its results can't help you?	**No. However, more ethnic mix in local population. Potential benefits depend on whether the reminder card is similar to that described in the study and the reasons for non-immunisation are similar.**

How great would the potential benefit of therapy actually be for your individual patient?

Method I: **f** **Your imm. rate is 82%, so risk of not being imm. is 18%**	(a) Risk of the outcome in your patient, relative to patients in the trial, expressed as a decimal: **18 / 33 = 0.55** (b) NNT/f = **8 / 0.55 = 14.5** (c) NNT for patients like yours **15**
Method II: **1 / (PEER × RRR)**	(a) Your patient's expected event rate if they received the control treatment: PEER: **18%** (b) 1 / (PEER × RRR) = 1/ **(0.18 × 0.36) = 15** (c) (NNT for patients like yours) **15**
Method III: **1 / PEER – (PEER × relative risk)**	(a) RR = 0.21/0.33 = **0.64** (b) 1 / PEER – (PEER × RR) = **15** (c) 1/0.18 – **(0.18 × 0.64) = 15** (d) NNT for patients like yours **15**

Are your patient's values and preferences satisfied by the regimen and its consequences?

Does your patient and you have a clear assessment of their values and preferences?	**Clear preference from public health point of view. Costs of changing card are small.**
Are they met by this regimen and its consequences?	**Determine locally.**

Additional notes

1. Method 3 for finding NNT : Look at reciprocal of absolute risk difference (ARR). Relative risk (RR) = EER/CER = 0.21 / 0.33 = 0.66. If your CER is 18% or 0.18, then with intervention, your EER is 0.66 × 0.18 = 0.115 or 11.5%
   ARR = 18% – 11.5% = 6.5%; NNT = 1/0.065 = 15
2. As control immunisation rates approach 100%, the relative risk is likely to change, and so estimate of NNT will change
3. In this scenario, the outcome measure (immunisation rate) is beneficial. Conventionally, we tend to look at adverse outcomes and risk reduction with experimental treatments, so in this scenario, look at the risk of *not* being immunised (100% – immunisation rate)

VACCINATION UPTAKE – CHANGES TO THE POSTAL REMINDER CARD CAN IMPROVE THE MEASLES IMMUNISATION UPTAKE

Appraised by O Duperrex and R Gilbert: 14 May 1999
Expiry date: March 2000.

Clinical Bottom Line
Changes to the postal reminder card based on a health belief model improved uptake of measles immunisation (NNT = 8 or a baseline risk of 33%).

Citation
Hawe P, McKenzie N and Scurry R (1998) Randomised controlled trial of the use of a modified postal reminder card on the uptake of measles vaccination. *Arch Dis Child* **79:** 136–140.

Clinical Question
In my community, would modification of the postal reminder card based on a health belief model, improve the immunisation uptake?

Search Terms
'vaccination / immunisation' and 'child' and 'uptake-rate' and 'postal-reminders' and 'randomized-controlled-trial'.

The Study
1 Randomised controlled trial with concealment of computer generated randomisation, objective and blind assessment of immunisation uptake and an intention-to-treat analysis.
2 The study patients: parents of children due for measles vaccination at 15 months were sent reminder cards 1 week before the next clinic.
3 Control group (N = 135): usual vaccination reminder card and a fixed appointment time (e.g. 2pm).
4 Experimental group (N = 124): personalised health belief model (HBM) card and an open appointment time (e.g. 2.00–3.30pm).

The Evidence

Outcome	Time to outcome	EER	CER	RRR	ARR	NNT
Not vaccinated	5 weeks	0.210	0.333	37%	0.124	8
95% confidence intervals				5–59%	0.016–0.22	4–63

Comments
1 No reliable information on comparability of groups at the start of the study.
2 Relative risk is likely to move nearer to 1.0 as vaccine uptake increases. In other words, the higher the uptake the more difficult it is to improve.
3 Potential benefits depend on type of reminder card currently used.

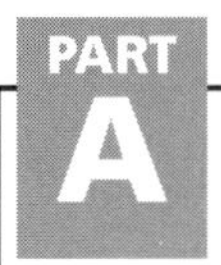

Critical appraisal of a clinical article about therapy

EBCH SESSION

1

SECTION 3

Therapy and introduction to CATS

Section 3: Croup

The practice nurse for a large health centre who is responsible for running the self-referral asthma clinic for children and young adults stops you (the GP) during the lunch break. She has just seen a 2-year-old child in the morning clinic with a barking cough and, from the description his mother gives, what sounds like inspiratory stridor during the previous night. She arranged for the child to be reviewed in your evening surgery. She poses the question, in children with mild to moderate croup, does nebulized budesonide decrease the risk of hospital admission compared with placebo? During her lunch break, she has a look for articles on the use of nebulized budesonide in croup on Medline (using Winspirs).

She presents you with her search strategy and a research article and asks whether you are going to give the child nebulized budesonide. By the time you see the child that evening, he has a barking cough, mild inspiratory stridor and a hoarse voice.

Decide:
1 Will you give the child nebulized budesonide?
2 Should you change local practice policy?

Search strategy for croup

Type in:
1 explode CROUP/ all subheadings
2 BUDESONIDE *
3 CLINICAL TRIAL IN PT*
4 #1 and #2 and #3

With this strategy, you find the article by Klassen *et al.* (*NEJM* 1994; **331:** 285–9.

Read the article and decide:
1 Is the evidence from this randomised trial valid?
2 If valid, is this evidence important?
3 If valid and important, can you apply this evidence in caring for your patient?

If you want to read some strategies for answering these sorts of questions, you could have a look at pp 91–6, 133–41 and 166–72 in *Evidence-based Medicine.*

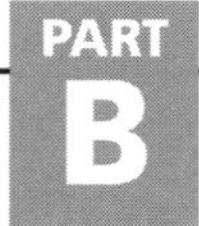

PART B How to use the CATMaker (optional)

If a CATMaker is provided with this package you will be shown how to use it to generate and save your own one page 'critically appraised topic' (CAT) from an article about therapy. The advantages of the CATMaker include its ability to calculate for you the clinically useful measures of the effects of therapy and their confidence intervals, and to save your critical appraisal for printing, sharing and storage.

The New England
Journal of Medicine

Volume 331 AUGUST 4, 1994 Number 5

NEBULIZED BUDESONIDE FOR CHILDREN WITH MILD-TO-MODERATE CROUP

TERRY P. KLASSEN, M.D., MARK E. FELDMAN, M.D., LISE K. WATTERS, M.D., TERESA SUTCLIFFE, R.N., AND PETER C. ROWE, M.D.

Abstract *Background.* Although recent evidence has strongly supported the use of glucocorticoid therapy in children hospitalized with croup, the benefit of this therapy in children with less severe croup has not been documented. This randomized, double-blind trial compared a nebulized glucocorticoid, budesonide, with placebo in outpatients with mild-to-moderate croup.

Methods. Children three months to five years of age were eligible for the study if their croup scores fell in the mild-to-moderate range (scores of 2 to 7 out of a possible 17). The patients were randomly assigned to receive either 2 mg (4 ml) of nebulized budesonide (27 children) or 4 ml of nebulized normal saline (27 children); they were then assessed hourly for up to four hours by investigators who were unaware of the assigned treatments.

Results. The median croup score at entry into the study was 4 in both groups. At the final study assessment, the median score was significantly lower in the budesonide group than in the placebo group (1 vs. 3, $P = 0.005$). The patients in the budesonide group were discharged from the emergency department significantly earlier than those in the placebo group ($P = 0.002$). One week after enrollment, 21 patients assigned to placebo had received dexamethasone, as compared with 15 patients assigned to budesonide ($P = 0.10$), and 7 patients assigned to placebo had been admitted to the hospital, as compared with 1 patient assigned to budesonide ($P = 0.05$).

Conclusions. We conclude that nebulized budesonide leads to a prompt and important clinical improvement in children with mild-to-moderate croup who come to the emergency department. (N Engl J Med 1994;331:285-9.)

CROUP (acute laryngotracheobronchitis) is a common cause of acute upper-airway obstruction in childhood, with an incidence of approximately 3 cases per 100 children less than six years of age. Up to 1.3 percent of affected children are hospitalized.[1] After several decades of debate,[2-11] the benefit of glucocorticoid therapy in patients hospitalized for croup has been firmly established by the results of four recent randomized clinical trials of intramuscular dexamethasone,[12,13] oral prednisolone,[14] and nebulized budesonide.[15]

Previous studies have not addressed whether the benefits of glucocorticoid therapy extend to children with milder disease, many of whom are evaluated in emergency departments. The argument against the routine use of glucocorticoids in outpatients has been that the majority of children with croup have self-limited illnesses.[16,17] It is not known, however, whether treatment at an early stage of the illness would reduce the severity of the clinical symptoms, prevent hospitalization or prolonged visits to the emergency department, and thereby both improve health outcomes and reduce costs.

We designed a randomized, placebo-controlled trial to determine whether nebulized budesonide leads to a clinically important improvement in respiratory symptoms within four hours for children with mild-to-moderate croup who come to the emergency department. Budesonide is a synthetic glucocorticoid with relatively strong topical antiinflammatory effects and low systemic activity as compared with beclomethasone.[18] Nebulized budesonide was selected for the study because it can be administered without the discomfort of intramuscular injection and because it begins to act as early as one hour after administration.[19]

METHODS

Selection of Patients

Patients coming to the emergency department at the Children's Hospital of Eastern Ontario between October 1, 1992, and October 15, 1993, were eligible for the study if they met the following criteria: an age of three months to five years; a syndrome consisting of hoarseness, inspiratory stridor, and barking cough; and a croup score of 2 or higher after breathing humidified oxygen for at least 15 minutes. Three research assistants trained by the investigators were on call to enroll patients in the study between 9 a.m. and midnight every day except holidays. Patients were excluded if they had been given a diagnosis of epiglottitis or chronic upper or lower airway disease (not including asthma), if corticosteroids had been administered within the preceding two weeks, or if they had severe croup. We defined children as having severe croup if their croup scores were 8 or higher or if they required treatment with racemic epinephrine immediately on arrival, as determined by the treating physician. The study was approved by the research ethics commit-

From the Department of Pediatrics, University of Ottawa, Ottawa, Ont. (T.P.K., L.K.W., T.S.); Scarborough Grace Hospital, Scarborough, Ont. (M.E.F.); and the Department of Pediatrics, Johns Hopkins University, Baltimore (P.C.R.). Address reprint requests to Dr. Rowe at the Department of Pediatrics, Johns Hopkins Hospital, 600 N. Wolfe St./Brady 212, Baltimore, MD 21287.

Supported by a grant (04410) from the Ontario Ministry of Health.

tee at the Children's Hospital of Eastern Ontario. Informed, written consent was obtained from all parents before the enrollment of patients.

Outcome Measures

All the patients underwent base-line clinical assessment by a research assistant, consisting of determination of the croup score,[20] respiratory rate, and heart rate while the patient breathed humidified oxygen or was inside a plastic enclosure (a croup tent). The croup score measured the degree of stridor (on a scale on which 0 denotes no stridor, 1 stridor audible with the stethoscope with the patient at rest, and 2 stridor audible without the stethoscope with the patient at rest), the severity of retraction of the intercostal and subcostal regions (0 denotes none, 1 mild, 2 moderate, and 3 severe), the entry of air into the lungs (0 denotes normal, 1 decreased, and 2 severely decreased), cyanosis (0 denotes none, 4 cyanosis with agitation, and 5 cyanosis at rest), and level of consciousness (0 denotes normal, and 5 altered).

In addition, the research assistants, parents, and treating physicians were asked at the end of the study period to rate independently whether the patient's condition had improved, remained the same, or worsened. This global assessment of change was then evaluated on a 15-point Likert scale ranging from −7 ("a very great deal worse") to +7 ("a very great deal better"), with 0 representing no change. The parents and the treating physicians were unaware of the patients' croup scores.

Study Design

Eligible patients were randomly assigned to receive a single dose containing either 2 mg (4 ml) of budesonide solution (Pulmicort, Astra, Pharma, Mississauga, Ont.) or 4 ml of 0.9 percent saline solution, administered by an updraft nebulizer with a continuous flow of oxygen at 5 to 6 liters per minute. Because budesonide is slightly opaque, the pharmacy provided both budesonide and normal saline in opaque brown syringes to ensure blinding. The research assistants then placed the study drug directly into an opaque nebulizer reservoir. Once nebulized, the study drugs were indistinguishable by sight and smell when tested before and during the study.

Randomization was performed in blocks of 10 by the pharmacy department, with a random-number table. Block randomization was used to ensure that there was an equal number of patients in the budesonide and placebo groups during the season when a respiratory virus was prevalent. The randomization list was kept concealed from the research assistants, parents, and emergency physicians and from the child's regular physician until the end of the trial. Thus, all treatment decisions during the week after enrollment were made by people unaware of the patient's treatment assignment.

The treating physicians followed the patients throughout the study period and were free to discharge them at any point if they deemed the patients clinically ready for discharge. The patients were given humidified oxygen through a large plastic tube (a mist stick) during the study period according to the protocol. To prevent the clinical trial from interfering with usual clinical practice, the treating physicians were free to use other interventions, such as racemic epinephrine or dexamethasone, or to place a patient in a croup tent for the delivery of humidified oxygen These interventions were defined as not being part of the study protocol. Once a patient received racemic epinephrine, measurements for that patient were not included in the hourly assessments. While the patients remained in the emergency department, they were assessed by the research assistant every hour for four hours, until the croup score was 1 or less, or until the treating physician considered the patient well enough to be sent home. The research assistant telephoned the family after one week to inquire about any further visits to doctors, further treatments, or hospitalizations.

Estimate of Sample Size

A two-point improvement in the croup score or a return of the score to 1 or less was considered to be clinically important and to constitute a response. We estimated that 40 percent of the patients assigned to placebo would have clinically important improvements, as compared with 70 percent of those assigned to budesonide. With a two-sided alpha level of 0.05 and 80 percent power, a sample containing 48 patients per group would be required.

During the trial, however, the clinicians in the emergency department came to consider the administration of dexamethasone to be the standard of care for children with croup that remained symptomatic after therapy with a mist stick. Because this change in clinical practice impaired our ability to recruit eligible patients and to evaluate the independent effect of budesonide, the study was stopped before the specified sample was reached and before the data were analyzed.

Statistical Analysis

The data were analyzed with SPSS/PC+ V4.01 software (SPSS, Chicago). Continuous data were analyzed with an independent two-tailed t-test when the data were parametric. Nonparametric data were analyzed with a Mann–Whitney U test. Categorical data were analyzed with the chi-square statistic or Fisher's exact test. Yates' continuity correction was used for two-by-two tables. Pearson's correlation coefficients were used to measure the association between the global assessment of change (on a 15-point Likert scale) and changes in the croup score, with a one-sided test for statistical significance. The survival analysis was performed with Kwikstat V3.01 (TexaSoft, Cedar Hill, Tex.), and differences between groups were tested with the Mantel–Haenszel test. Agreement between observers was measured by the kappa statistic with quadratic weights with use of PC-Agree software (McMaster University, Hamilton, Ont.).

Results

Characteristics of the Patients

During the study period, 390 patients had a diagnosis of croup on discharge from the emergency department. Of these patients, 163 presented at times when the study team was not on call, and in 24 additional cases the emergency department failed to contact the study team. A further 146 patients did not meet the eligibility criteria for the study because they had croup that was too mild (83 patients), did not meet the age requirement (31 patients), did not meet our definition of croup (16 patients), had croup that was too severe (5 patients), had epiglottitis (3 patients), had previous upper airway disease (2 patients), or had recently been treated with steroids (1 patient). The parents of the remaining 57 patients were approached about participation in the study, and 54 agreed on behalf of their children.

Twenty-seven patients were randomly assigned to the budesonide group and 27 to the placebo group. Table 1 shows that most base-line demographic and clinical variables were evenly distributed between the two groups, except for temperature and the duration of cough, differences that would have favored the placebo group.

Variation between Observers

The research assistants and physician investigators rated the croup scores of 12 patients concurrently to measure interobserver reliability. The weighted kappa statistic (±SE) was 0.95±0.02, indicating excellent agreement.

Outcome Variables

As compared with the patients assigned to placebo, the patients treated with budesonide had significantly lower croup scores at the final study assessment (median, 3 vs. 1; P = 0.005) (Table 2). There were

Table 1. Characteristics of Patients at Entry into the Study.*

Variable	Budesonide (N = 27)	Placebo (N = 27)	P Value
Male sex (no.)	17	20	0.56
Age (yr)	1.8±1.2	2.2±1.4	0.26
No. with preceding upper respiratory infection	18	16	0.78
Duration of cough (days)	1.4±0.9	0.9±0.9	0.03
No. with previous croup	7	8	1.0
No. with previous asthma	4	5	0.57
Duration of mist therapy before study (min)	73±37	62±33	0.25
Temperature (°C)	38.2±0.8	37.6±1.2	0.04
Croup score†	4 (3, 5)	4 (3, 5)	0.13
Heart rate (beats/min)	151±22	147±26	0.61
Respiratory rate (breaths/min)	41±14	36±12	0.13

*Plus-minus values are means ±SD.

†Values are expressed as medians, followed in parentheses by the 25th and 75th percentiles.

no significant differences between the groups in heart rate or respiratory rate at the final study assessment (Table 2). When the a priori definition of response was used, at four hours 19 of the budesonide group had a response (70 percent), as compared with 10 of the placebo group (37 percent) (P = 0.03).

Table 3 shows that the global assessment of change by the research assistants, parents, and treating physicians significantly favored the patients assigned to budesonide. The condition of only one patient in the budesonide group was found to have worsened after the assessment period. Table 3 also shows a significant correlation between the independent global assessments by different groups of observers and the changes in the croup scores from the beginning to the end of the study period.

At the end of the four-hour assessment period, 14 patients remained in the budesonide group, whereas the other 13 had improved enough to be discharged from the study. Fifteen patients remained in the placebo group; of the remaining 12, 8 had improved enough to be discharged home, 1 was withdrawn from the study by a parent (upset because the child was not improving; the child's croup score was 5), and 3 were withdrawn because of substantial worsening of croup (2 received racemic epinephrine and 1 was admitted to the hospital). Among those who remained in the emergency department for the four-hour evaluation, the patients assigned to budesonide had significantly lower median croup scores (2.5, vs. 4.0 for the placebo group; P = 0.05).

Other Interventions

Patients received other interventions at the discretion of their treating physicians, who remained unaware of the treatment assignments. Two patients in the placebo group received racemic epinephrine, as compared with none of the patients in the budesonide group (P = 0.49). There was no difference between the groups in the proportion of patients for whom a croup tent was ordered (P = 1.0). Six patients in the budesonide group (22 percent) received dexamethasone during the study period, as compared with eight of those in the placebo group (30 percent) (P = 0.75). The mean (±SD) interval before the administration of dexamethasone did not differ significantly between groups (budesonide, 148±35 minutes; placebo, 122±34; P = 0.19).

In addition to the patients who received dexamethasone in the emergency department during the study period, 9 patients assigned to budesonide (33 percent) and 11 patients assigned to placebo (41 percent) received dexamethasone before discharge from the emergency department (P = 0.34).

Follow-up

A survival analysis of the time until patients were sent home from the emergency department or the holding unit revealed a significantly earlier discharge for patients treated with budesonide than for those receiving placebo (P = 0.002) (Fig. 1). By the end of the four-hour study period, 12 patients in the budesonide group (44 percent) were sent home, as compared with 6 patients in the placebo group (22 percent). Six patients assigned to placebo (22 percent) were admitted to the hospital for a median stay of two days (range, one to five), as compared with one patient assigned to budesonide (4 percent), who remained in the hospital two days.

At the one-week follow-up, family members of all the patients in the trial were contacted by telephone. Ten patients in each group had visited a doctor; these physicians did not know which study treatment the patient had received. One of the patients in the placebo group who was not initially admitted to a hospital required hospital admission for three days starting two days after discharge from the emergency department, and two patients in the placebo group received dexamethasone in the week after discharge from the emergency department, as compared with none in the budesonide group. From the start of the study until the end of the first week, 21 patients assigned to placebo (78 percent) had received dexamethasone, as compared with 15 patients assigned to budesonide (56 percent) (P = 0.10). By the end of the first week, seven patients in the placebo group (26 percent) had been admitted, as compared with one patient in the budesonide group (4 percent) (P = 0.05).

Possible Adverse Effects of Treatment

No adverse events were noted in the budesonide group. No patient in that group had clinical deterioration, either in the emergency department or after

Table 2. Outcome Variables at the Final Study Assessment.*

Variable	Budesonide (N = 27)	Placebo (N = 27)	P Value
Croup score†	1 (0, 3)	3 (1, 5)	0.005
Respiratory rate (breaths/min)	32±7	33±10	0.5
Heart rate (beats/min)	128±20	138±21	0.03

*Plus-minus values are means ±SD.

†Values are expressed as medians, followed in parentheses by the 25th and 75th percentiles.

discharge. One patient in the placebo group had a burning sensation on the face.

Discussion

This randomized, controlled trial has demonstrated an important clinical benefit of budesonide treatment in patients with mild-to-moderate croup. The improvement associated with budesonide was reflected in lower croup scores, improved global ratings by independent observers, earlier discharge from the emergency department, and a lower rate of hospital admissions and other interventions by physicians who were unaware of the treatment assignment.

A useful index of therapeutic benefit is the number of patients who would need to be treated by an intervention for one patient to have the outcome event of interest.[21] On the basis of the data from this trial, for example, five patients with croup scores of 2 to 7 would need to be treated with nebulized budesonide for one hospitalization to be prevented. For one patient to have a clinically important response under our definition, three patients would need to be treated with budesonide. These results indicate the potential for a substantial reduction in health care expenditures for croup, because the cost of a single dose of nebulized budesonide is dwarfed by the cost of even a two-day admission to the hospital.

The demonstration that budesonide has a therapeutic effect within four hours in children with mild-to-moderate croup is consistent with observations from other studies and studies in animals.[22,23] Among patients hospitalized for croup who were assessed with a clinical scoring system similar to the one we used, Husby and colleagues observed a significant improvement two hours after administering 2 mg of nebulized budesonide.[15]

When a clinical score is used as an outcome measure, it should be valid, reliable, and responsive to important changes in clinical status.[24] These methodologic properties of the croup score have received little attention in the past, although the score has been used

Table 3. Global Assessments of Change in the Patients' Condition at the End of the Study Period.

Observer and Group	Patient's Condition			P Value*	Correlation with Change in Croup Score
	Worse	No Change	Better		
	no. of patients				
Research assistant					
Budesonide	1	5	21		
Placebo	7	6	14	0.05	0.76 (P = 0.001)
Parent†					
Budesonide	0	7	19		
Placebo	4	5	15	0.10	0.56 (P = 0.001)
Treating physician†					
Budesonide	0	5	16		
Placebo	7	3	13	0.03	0.51 (P = 0.001)

*For the comparison of the global assessments of change in the two groups, by the chi-square test (three-by-two table).

†Fewer than 27 patients are shown for the groups in this category because the observer was not always available at the end of the assessment period.

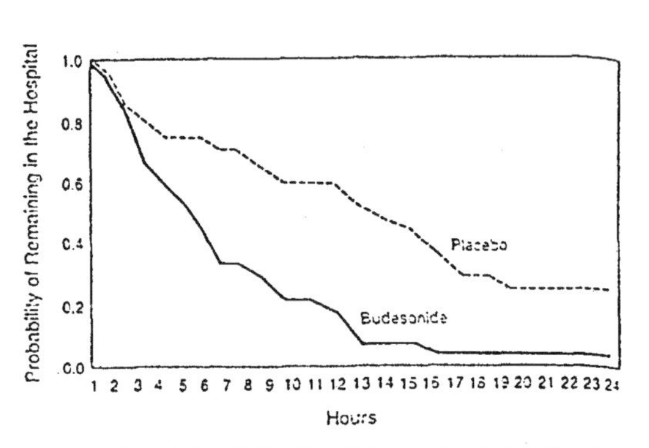

Figure 1. Cumulative Probability of Remaining in the Hospital (Ward, Emergency Department, or Holding Unit) after Treatment with Budesonide or Placebo.

The survival curves were compared by the Mantel–Haenszel test (chi-square with 1 df = 9.35, P = 0.002).

as the primary outcome measure in most clinical trials in children with this condition. As far as we are aware, the only available validation study showed that the croup score correlated with changes in the diameter of the tracheal lumen before and after treatment with racemic epinephrine in 12 children whose mean croup score before treatment was 4.[25] Our study has generated data on both validity and responsiveness by showing that the croup score correlates with the global judgments of three groups of independent observers who have different perspectives on the patient.

One other aspect of the study methods deserves comment. Although dexamethasone treatment had the potential to interfere with assessment of the independent effect of budesonide, by one week after enrollment 78 percent of the placebo group had received dexamethasone, as compared with 56 percent of the budesonide group. Only those in the placebo group were treated with racemic epinephrine. The overall effect of both interventions would have been to reduce the likelihood of detecting the observed difference between the patients in the budesonide group and those in the placebo group.

Past admonitions against the routine use of glucocorticoids in patients with croup have stressed the potential for infrequent but serious gastrointestinal hemorrhage and other adverse effects after dexamethasone therapy.[16,26] To some observers, these risks seemed unnecessarily large for children with mild or moderate croup in whom recovery was virtually assured, albeit occasionally after a brief hospitalization. Because budesonide does not carry a risk of either gastrointestinal hemorrhage or painful injection, the demonstration of its efficacy in mild-to-moderate croup shifts the risk–benefit ratio in favor of treatment. Further study will help determine whether giving budesonide alone at an early phase of the illness has a sustained effect on the course of croup and whether children with croup are most responsive to glucocorticoid therapy at an early point in the illness, before excessive subglottic edema has developed.

Glucocorticoids should be used with caution in patients with preexisting immunodeficiency, recent exposure to varicella, or possible tuberculosis. When used in previously healthy children with croup, however, glucocorticoids given orally or parenterally have had few important adverse effects.[27,28] The systemic toxic effects of inhaled steroids should be even more limited than those associated with the oral or parenteral forms. Although our study had 100 percent follow-up at one week, we would emphasize that our sample was not large enough for rare side effects to be identified.[29]

We conclude that nebulized budesonide is an effective initial therapy for children with mild-to-moderate croup who come to the emergency department and remain symptomatic after mist therapy. With its rapid action and prolonged effect, budesonide may be a valuable agent for inhibiting the subglottic inflammatory edema that contributes to stridor in children with croup.

We are indebted to Pat Harman and Joanne Momy for their tireless work as research assistants, to Colline Blanchard for randomization and drug preparation, to Dr. Marilyn Li and all the pediatricians and nurses in the Emergency Department for help in recruiting patients, to Dr. Martin Osmond and Grace Dueck for their critical review of an earlier version of this manuscript, and to Robert Stenstrom for assistance with the early development of this project.

References

1. Denny FW, Murphy TF, Clyde WA Jr, Collier AM, Henderson FW. Croup: an 11-year study in a pediatric practice. Pediatrics 1983;71:871-6.
2. [illegible], Nilsson G, Torbjär J-E. The effect of corticosteroids in the treatment of pseudo-croup. Acta Otolaryngol Suppl 1960;158:62-71.
3. Novik A. Corticosteroid treatment of non-diphtheritic croup. Acta Otolaryngol Suppl 1960:158:20-3.
4. Eden AN, Larkin VP. Corticosteroid treatment of croup. Pediatrics 1964;33:768-9.
5. Sussman S, Grossman M, Magoffin R, Schieble J. Dexamethasone (16 alpha-methyl, 9 alpha-fluoroprednisolone) in obstructive respiratory tract infections in children: a controlled study. Pediatrics 1964;34:851-5.
6. Skowron PN, Turner JA, McNaughton GA. The use of corticosteroid (dexamethasone) in the treatment of acute laryngotracheitis. Can Med Assoc J 1966;94:528-31.
7. Eden AN, Kaufman A, Yu R. Corticosteroids and croup: controlled double-blind study. JAMA 1967;200:403-4.
8. James JA. Dexamethasone in croup: a controlled study. Am J Dis Child 1969:117:511-6.
9. Leipzig B, Oski FA, Cummings CW, Stockman JA, Swender P. A prospective randomized study to determine the efficacy of steroids in treatment of croup. J Pediatr 1979;94:194-6.
10. Muhlendahl KE, Kahn D, Spohr HL, Dressler F. Steroid treatment of pseudo-croup. Helv Paediatr Acta 1982;37:431-6.
11. Koren G, Frand M, Barzilay Z, MacLeod SM. Corticosteroid treatment of laryngotracheitis v spasmodic croup in children. Am J Dis Child 1983;137:941-4.
12. Super DM, Cartelli NA, Brooks LJ, Lembo RM, Kumar ML. A prospective randomized double-blind study to evaluate the effect of dexamethasone in acute laryngotracheitis. J Pediatr 1989;115:323-9.
13. Kuusela AL, Vesikari T. A randomized double-blind, placebo-controlled trial of dexamethasone and racemic epinephrine in the treatment of croup. Acta Paediatr Scand 1988;77:99-104.
14. Tibballs J, Shann FA, Landau LI. Placebo-controlled trial of prednisolone in children intubated for croup. Lancet 1992;340:745-8.
15. Husby S, Agertoft L, Mortensen S, Pedersen S. Treatment of croup with nebulised steroid (budesonide): a double blind, placebo controlled study. Arch Dis Child 1993;68:352-5.
16. Smith DS. Corticosteroids in croup: a chink in the ivory tower? J Pediatr 1989;115:256-7.
17. Steroids and croup. Lancet 1989;2:1134-6.
18. Johansson SA, Andersson KE, Brattsand R, Gruvstad E, Hedner P. Topical and systemic glucocorticoid potencies of budesonide and beclomethasone in man. Eur J Clin Pharmacol 1982;22:523-9.
19. Ellul-Micallef R, Johansson SA. Acute dose-response studies in bronchial asthma with a new corticosteroid, budesonide. Br J Clin Pharmacol 1983;15:419-22.
20. Westley CR, Cotton EK, Brooks JG. Nebulized racemic epinephrine by IPPB for the treatment of croup: a double-blind study. Am J Dis Child 1978;132:484-7.
21. Laupacis A, Sackett DL, Roberts RS. An assessment of clinically useful measures of the consequences of treatment. N Engl J Med 1988;318:1728-33.
22. Miller-Larsson A, Brattsand R. Topical anti-inflammatory activity of the glucocorticoid budesonide on airway mucosa: evidence for a "hit and run" type of activity. Agents Actions 1990;29:127-9.
23. Erlansson M, Svensjo E, Bergqvist D. Leukotriene B4-induced permeability increase in postcapillary venules and its inhibition by three different antiinflammatory drugs. Inflammation 1989;13:693-705.
24. Guyatt GH, Kirshner B, Jaeschke R. Measuring health status: what are the necessary measurement properties? J Clin Epidemiol 1992;45:1341-5.
25. Corkey CWB, Barker GA, Edmonds JF, Mok PM, Newth CJL. Radiographic tracheal diameter measurements in acute infectious croup: an objective scoring system. Crit Care Med 1981;9:587-90.
26. Cherry JD. The treatment of croup: continued controversy due to failure of recognition of historic, ecologic, etiologic and clinical perspectives. J Pediatr 1979;94:352-4.
27. Skolnik NS. Treatment of croup: a critical review. Am J Dis Child 1989;143:1045-9.
28. Kairys SW, Olmstead EM, O'Connor GT. Steroid treatment of laryngotracheitis: a meta-analysis of the evidence from randomized trials. Pediatrics 1989;83:683-93.
29. Lentner C, ed. Geigy scientific tables. Vol. 2. Introduction to statistics, statistical tables, mathematical formulae. 8th rev. enl. ed. Basel, Switzerland: Ciba-Geigy, 1982:26-9.

THERAPY WORKSHEET: 1 of 2

Clinical question:

Are the results of this single preventive or therapeutic trial valid?

Was the assignment of patients to treatments randomised?
Was the randomisation list concealed?

Were all patients who entered the trial accounted for at its conclusion?
Were they analysed in the groups to which they were randomised?

Were patients and clinicians kept 'blind' to which treatment was being received?

Aside from the experimental treatment, were the groups treated equally?

Were the groups similar at the start of the trial?

Are the valid results of this randomised trial important?

SAMPLE CALCULATIONS (see pp 134–40 of *Evidence-based Medicine*)

Occurrence of diabetic neuropathy		Relative risk reduction (RRR)	Absolute risk reduction (ARR)	Number needed to treat (NNT)
Usual insulin control event rate (CER)	Intensive insulin experimental event rate (EER)	$\frac{CER - EER}{CER}$	CER – EER	1 / ARR
9.6%	2.8%	$\frac{9.6\% - 2.8\%}{9.6\%}$ = 71%	9.6% – 2.8% = 6.8%	1 / 6.8% = 15 pts

95% confidence interval (CI) on an NNT = 1 / (limits on the CI of its ARR) =

$$+/-1.96\sqrt{\frac{CER \times (1-CER)}{\#\text{ of control pts}} + \frac{EER \times (1-EER)}{\#\text{ of exper. pts}}} = +/-1.96\sqrt{\frac{0.096 \times 0.904}{730} + \frac{0.028 \times 0.972}{711}} = \pm 2.4\%$$

YOUR CALCULATIONS

		Relative risk reduction (RRR)	Absolute risk reduction (ARR)	Number needed to treat (NNT)
CER	EER	$\frac{CER - EER}{CER}$	CER – EER	1 / ARR

Can you apply this valid, important evidence about a treatment in caring for your patient?

Do these results apply to your patient?

Is your patient so different from those in the trial that its results can't help you?

How great would the potential benefit of therapy actually be for your individual patient?

Method I: **f**	(a) Risk of the outcome in your patient, relative to patients in the trial, expressed as a decimal:_____ (b) NNT/f = ___/___ = (c) NNT for patients like yours
Method II: **1 / (PEER × RRR)**	(a) Your patient's expected event rate if they received the control treatment: PEER:______ (b) 1 / (PEER × RRR) = 1/______ = _______ (c) NNT for patients like yours
Method III: **1 / PEER – (PEER × Relative risk)**	(a) Your patient's expected event rate if they received the control treatment: PEER:______ (b) Relative risk – EER/CER =______ (c) 1 / PEER – (PEER × Relative risk) =______ (d) NNT for patients like yours

Are your patient's values and preferences satisfied by the regimen and its consequences?

Does your patient and you have a clear assessment of their values and preferences?

Are they met by this regimen and its consequences?

Additional notes

Clinical question: In children of mild-to-moderate croup does nubulized budesonide compared to placebo reduce the risk of hospital admission?

Are the results of this single preventive or therapeutic trial valid?

Was the assignment of patients to treatments randomised? Was the randomisation list concealed?	**Yes, and randomisation performed by pharmacy was concealed.**
Were all patients who entered the trial accounted for at its conclusion? Were they analysed in the groups to which they were randomised?	**Yes.** **Yes.**
Were patients and clinicians kept 'blind' to which treatment was being received?	**Yes. Both budesonide and placebo were given in opaque chambers.**
Aside from the experimental treatment, were the groups treated equally?	**Yes.**
Were the groups similar at the start of the trial?	**Yes, more or less. Slightly longer duration of cough and higher temperature in experimental group.**

Are the valid results of this randomised trial important?

SAMPLE CALCULATIONS (*see* pp 134–40 of *Evidence-based Medicine*)

Occurrence of diabetic neuropathy		**Relative risk reduction (RRR)**	**Absolute risk reduction (ARR)**	**Number needed to treat (NNT)**
Usual insulin control event rate (CER)	Intensive insulin experimental event rate (EER)	$\frac{\text{CER} - \text{EER}}{\text{CER}}$	CER – EER	1 / ARR
9.6%	2.8%	$\frac{9.6\% - 2.8\%}{9.6\%}$ = 71%	9.6% – 2.8% = 6.8%	1 / 6.8% = 15 pts

95% confidence interval (CI) on an NNT = 1 / (limits on the CI of its ARR) =

$$+/-1.96\sqrt{\frac{\text{CER}\times(1-\text{CER})}{\#\text{ of control pts}}+\frac{\text{EER}\times(1-\text{EER})}{\#\text{ of exper. pts}}} = +/-1.96\sqrt{\frac{0.096\times0.904}{730}+\frac{0.028\times0.972}{711}} = \pm2.4\%$$

YOUR CALCULATIONS

Hospital admission		**Relative risk reduction (RRR)**	**Absolute risk reduction (ARR)**	**Number needed to treat (NNT)**
CER	EER	$\frac{\text{CER} - \text{EER}}{\text{CER}}$	CER – EER	1 / ARR
1/27 = .04	**7/27 = .26**	**0.85**	**0.22**	**5**

Can you apply this valid, important evidence about a treatment in caring for your patient?	
Do these results apply to your patient?	
Is your patient so different from those in the trial that its results can't help you?	**No. Patient in the scenario has a croup score 2–3, similar to patients in the trial. Assume baseline risk of hospital admission is 5%.**
How great would the potential benefit of therapy actually be for your individual patient?	
Method I: **f**	(a) Risk of the outcome in your patient, relative to patients in the trial. Expressed as a decimal: 0.2 (b) NNT/f = 5 / 0.2 = 25 (c) NNT for patients like yours = 25
Method II: **1 / (PEER × RRR)**	(a) Your patient's expected event rate if they received the control treatment: PEER: 5% (b) 1 / (PEER × RRR) = 1/.05 × .85 = 24 (c) NNT for patients like yours = 24
Method III: **1 / PEER – (PEER × Relative risk)**	(a) Your patient's expected event rate if they received the control treatment: PEER: 5% (b) Relative risk – EER/CER = 0.15 (c) 1 / PEER – (PEER × Relative Risk) = 24 (d) NNT for patients like yours = 24
Are your patient's values and preferences satisfied by the regimen and its consequences?	
Do your patient and you have a clear assessment of their values and preferences?	**Consider inconvenience and cost of nebuliser versus hospital admissions saved.**
Are they met by this regimen and its consequences?	**Yes, probably.**

Additional notes

1. The study includes a mix of mild-to-moderate croup. In primary care, mild cases will predominate and the treatment effect may differ. Caution in applying these results to primary care.
2. You may wish to look for evidence on oral steroids such as dexamethasone.

CROUP – NEBULIZED BUDESONIDE REDUCES HOSPITAL ADMISSION IN CHILDREN WITH MILD-TO-MODERATE CROUP

Appraised by O Duperrex and R Gilbert: 14 May 1999
Expiry date: March 2000.

Clinical Bottom Line

Nebulized budesonide compared with placebo reduces hospital admission and improves symptoms in children with mild to moderate croup.

Citation

Klassen TP, Feldman ME and Watters LK (1994) Nebulized budesonide for children with mild to moderate croup. *NEJM* **331**(5): 285–89.

Clinical Question

In children with mild-to-moderate croup does nebulized budesonide compared with placebo reduce the risk of hospital admission?

Search Terms

'explode CROUP/all subheadings' and 'BUDESONIDE*' and 'CLINICAL TRIAL IN PT*'.

The Study

1 Randomised, controlled trial of children with croup score of 2–7 (out of possible 17) seen in A&E department.
2 Randomisation was concealed and children, parents and clinicians were blind to treatment.
3 They performed an intention to treat analysis.
4 Control group (N = 27; 27 analysed) : 4 ml nebulized normal saline.
5 Experimental group (N = 27; 27 analysed) : 4 ml nebulized budesonide (2 mg).

The Evidence

Admission one week later

EER	CER	ARR (95% CI)	NNT (95% CI)
1/27 = 0.4	7/27 = 0.26	0.22 (0.042 – 0.402)	5 (2 – 24)

Mean 2 point reduction in croup score in treatment group ($p<.05$)

Comments

1 The small number of patients studied produces wide confidence intervals.
2 Watch for more recent studies on this topic.

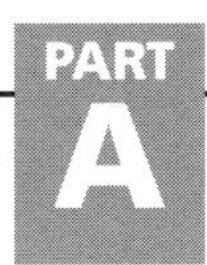

Critical appraisal of a clinical article about diagnosis

EBCH SESSION

2

SECTION 1

Diagnosis and asking answerable clinical questions

Section 1: Clinical examination for heart defects in Down's syndrome

You are the midwife looking after a mother and her newborn baby, who has marked characteristics of Down's syndrome. The family understand the likely diagnosis and, as the baby appears well at 2 days of age, are keen to go home and await the results of the chromosome analysis. The baby has been examined by the consultant paediatrician who found no abnormal signs on clinical examination or chest X-ray, and referred the baby for echo-cardiography at the teaching hospital 50 miles away. However, the family are reluctant to undergo further tests at present and ask whether it would do any harm to wait a few months before seeing the paediatric cardiologist. You formulate the question, in babies with Down's syndrome, how useful are the clinical examination, chest X-ray and the ECG in predicting the risk of congenital heart disease? Fortunately, Medline is accessible from the ward computer and you do a literature search and find the enclosed paper before the paediatrician arrives to discharge the baby.

What is your assessment of the risks for the baby?

Search strategy for clinical examination for heart defects in Down's syndrome

Type in:
1 down syndrome/
2 exp heart defects, congenital/
3 #1 and # 2
4 exp diagnosis/
5 #3 and #4
6 "sensitivity and specificity"/
7 #5 and #6

With this strategy, you find the article by Tubman *et al.* (*BMJ* 1991; **302:** 1425–7)

Read this article and decide:
1 Are the results of this diagnostic article valid?
2 Are the valid results of this diagnostic study important?
3 Can you apply this valid, important evidence about a diagnostic test in caring for your patient?

If you want to read some strategies for answering these sorts of questions, you could have a look at pp 81–4, 118–28 and 159–63 in *Evidence-based Medicine*.

PART B

Asking answerable clinical questions

We will illustrate the importance, strategies, and tactics of formulating clinical questions and work with you on the 3–4 parts of the question.

Participants will break up into groups of two, discuss patients they cared for in the previous week, and generate questions they think are important concerning their patients' therapy, diagnosis and prognosis.

In larger groups, we will review and refine the questions, and then keep track of them as possible questions to use in later sessions devoted to searching for the best evidence.

PAPERS

Congenital heart disease in Down's syndrome: two year prospective early screening study

T R J Tubman, M D Shields, B G Craig, H C Mulholland, N C Nevin

Abstract

Objective—To determine the effectiveness of clinical examination, chest radiography, and electrocardiography compared with echocardiography in detecting congenital heart disease early in the life of children with Down's syndrome.

Design—Prospective two year screening survey.

Setting—Regional paediatric cardiology service, Northern Ireland.

Patients—81 newborn infants with Down's syndrome born in Northern Ireland between November 1987 and November 1989.

Interventions—Clinical examination, chest radiography, and electrocardiography soon after birth followed by cross sectional Doppler echocardiography.

Main outcome measures—Diagnostic ability of clinical examination, radiography, and electrocardiography compared with echocardiographic findings.

Results—34 babies had congenital heart disease detected by echocardiography (13 had atrioventricular septal defects, seven secundum atrial septal defects, six a solitary patent ductus arteriosus, five isolated ventricular septal defects, and three combinations of heart defects). Individual examination methods were insensitive (the sensitivity of clinical examination was 0·53, of radiography 0·44, and of electrocardiography 0·41) but highly specific (the specificity of clinical examination was 0·94, of radiography 0·98, and of electrocardiography 1·0), although sensitivity improved when the three techniques were combined (the sensitivity was 0·71, the specificity 0·91).

Conclusion—Echocardiography performed early in life can detect congenital heart disease that might otherwise be missed. Early detection may help prevent complications such as pulmonary vascular disease that may adversely affect the outcome of cardiac surgery.

Cardiac Unit, Royal Belfast Hospital for Sick Children, Belfast
T R J Tubman, MRCP, *paediatric registrar*
M D Shields, MRCP, *paediatric senior registrar*
B G Craig, MRCP, *consultant paediatric cardiologist*
H C Mulholland, FRCPED, *consultant paediatric cardiologist*

Northern Ireland Genetics Service, Belfast City Hospital, Belfast
N C Nevin, FRCPED, *professor of medical genetics*

Correspondence to: Dr T R J Tubman, Neonatal Unit, Royal Maternity Hospital, Belfast BT12 6BB.

BMJ 1991;302:1425-7

Introduction

Down's syndrome (trisomy 21) is the commonest cause of mental handicap in Northern Ireland.[1] Its association with congenital heart disease is well known, the reported incidence being 40-60%.[2-4] Congenital heart disease contributes significantly to the morbidity and mortality of children with Down's syndrome, who may develop congestive heart failure, pulmonary vascular disease, pneumonia, or failure to thrive. In the first few days of life symptoms or signs may be absent or minimal despite the presence of significant congenital heart disease. For some time we have thought that parents of some children with Down's syndrome and congenital heart disease (particularly atrioventricular septal defects) have been reassured initially by paediatricians that their child's heart is probably normal until sequelae such as pulmonary vascular disease have become evident. We therefore undertook a prospective study to screen for congenital heart disease in babies with Down's syndrome at or as soon after birth as possible. We determined the incidence of congenital heart disease in such babies born in Northern Ireland and the incidences of specific forms of cardiac defect. We also compared the effectiveness of the current practice of clinical examination, chest radiography, and electrocardiography with screening by cross sectional echocardiography.

Patients and methods

We prospectively examined all new babies with Down's syndrome who were born in Northern Ireland within a two year period from November 1987 to November 1989. The diagnosis in all babies was later confirmed by chromosomal analysis. All consultant paediatricians and obstetricians in Northern Ireland were asked to notify the Regional Paediatric Cardiology Service of new cases of Down's syndrome at or as soon after birth as possible. Clinical findings suggestive of congenital heart disease including cyanosis, tachypnoea, an abnormal precordial impulse, or a murmur were recorded by the referring clinician; chest radiography and electrocardiography were performed when possible.

Babies were then referred to the regional paediatric cardiology unit for further clinical examination and cross sectional Doppler echocardiography. If a chest radiograph or electrocardiogram had not been taken by the referring hospital the salient procedure was then performed. In several cases (mainly because of geographical distance) echocardiography could not be performed within the first few days of life; under these circumstances babies were seen at one of four paediatric cardiology clinics held monthly in peripheral district general hospitals. Thus newborn babies with Down's syndrome could be seen within the first month of life and in most cases within the first few days of life for a full cardiological assessment.

In addition, monthly returns of every new case of Down's syndrome confirmed by chromosomal analysis were supplied by the Northern Ireland Genetics Service. These were cross checked against clinical referrals; the parents or general practitioners of missing babies were contacted by telephone and arrangements made to examine these babies as soon as possible. In general, babies born in hospitals with no on site paediatric service were more likely to be picked up in this way.

Cross sectional Doppler echocardiography was taken as the "gold standard" for detecting congenital heart defects and the results from it were compared with those from standard methods of examination—that is, clinical examination, chest radiography, and electrocardiography—both separately and collectively. In a few babies echocardiography detected a small patent ductus arteriosus or a patent foramen ovale within the first few days of life. As these findings could have been a part of the normal neonatal transitional circulation, reassessment was made one month later for a definitive diagnosis.

Data were analysed to determine sensitivity, specificity, and positive and negative predictive values[5] for each of the clinical methods of screening used alone and in combination and were compared with the results for echocardiography.

Results

INCIDENCE OF CONGENITAL HEART DISEASE

In the two year study period a total of 81 babies were referred either by clinicians (69) or by the genetics service (12) and screened for congenital heart disease. Fifty three were boys and 28 girls. There were 53 847 live births in Nothern Ireland during this period, giving an annual incidence of 1·50 per 1000 live births. Sixty one babies were examined by echocardiography in the first two weeks of life and 74 before 3 months of age.

Thirty four babies had congenital heart disease detectable by cross sectional echocardiography. The proportion of affected boys and girls was similar (40% males *v* 46% females). Of the affected babies, 13 had atrioventricular septal defects, seven secundum atrial septal defects, six a large solitary patent ductus arteriosus, and five isolated ventricular septal defects. Three babies had a combination of heart defects—namely, atrioventricular septal defect with coarctation of aorta and patent ductus arteriosus; secundum atrial septal defect with ventricular septal defect and a right sided overriding aorta (but no pulmonary stenosis); and ventricular septal defect with secundum atrial septal defect and mild pulmonary valvar stenosis. Eight of the 13 atrioventricular septal defects had an associated patent ductus arteriosus, usually with detectable left to right flow. Similarly, three of the seven secundum atrial septal defects had an associated patent ductus arteriosus.

SCREENING

Table I shows the diagnostic ability of the three clinical tests alone and in combination.

Clinical examination—Of the 81 babies examined, 21 had abnormal clinical findings suggestive of congenital heart disease. Heart disease was confirmed in 18 of them, but the remaining three had structurally normal hearts (two had "cyanosis" due to polycythaemia and persistent fetal circulation and one had an innocent systolic murmur). Of the 60 babies thought by referring clinicians to have no heart disease, 16 had structural defects detected by echocardiography (five had atrioventricular septal defects, six secundum atrial septal defects, three ventricular septal defects, one had a patent ductus arteriosus, and one a combination of defects). Five of these babies had more subtle clinical signs, such as an accentuated pulmonary second sound, detected on re-examination by cardiologists (two had atrioventricular septal defects, one secundum atrial septal defect, one a patent ductus arteriosus, and one a combination of defects). Thus clinical examination by referring clinicians had a sensitivity of 0·53 and a specificity of 0·94.

Chest radiography—Sixteen babies had an initial chest radiograph reported as abnormal; on re-examination one of these was suggestive of transient tachypnoea of the newborn rather than pulmonary oedema. Nineteen babies had a normal chest radiograph but had a structural abnormality diagnosed by echocardiography (three had atrioventricular septal defects, five ventricular septal defects, six had secundum atrial septal defects, four a patent ductus arteriosus, and one a combination of defects). Compared with echocardiography, chest radiography had a sensitivity of 0·44 and a specificity of 0·98.

Electrocardiography—Seventy nine of the 81 babies were examined by electrocardiography. In one baby the heart condition had already been diagnosed by echocardiography; the other baby, a preterm of 28 weeks' gestation, died before electrocardiography could be performed but had a chest radiograph and an echocardiogram. Both babies had congenital heart disease (one had an atrioventricular septal defect, the other a secundum atrial septal defect). Sixty six babies had a normal electrocardiogram, but 19 of them had congenital heart disease (two had atrioventricular septal defects, four ventricular septal defects, five secundum atrial septal defects, five a patent ductus arteriosus, and three a combination of defects). Of the 13 babies with an abnormal electrocardiogram—that is, an abnormal QRS axis or evidence of ventricular hypertrophy—10 had atrioventricular septal defects, one a ventricular septal defect, one a secundum atrial septal defect, and one a large patent ductus arteriosus. There were no false positive electrocardiograms. Thus electrocardiography alone had a much higher specificity and positive predictive value (both 1·0) than the two other methods of screening.

The three techniques combined—When the three diagnostic procedures were combined, with at least one of them giving a positive result, sensitivity was greater than when any one test was used alone, though specificity was reduced because of four false positive results (table II). Despite the increased sensitivity, 10 babies had heart disease which would not have been detected without echocardiography (two had atrioventricular septal defects, five secundum atrial septal defects, two ventricular septal defects, and one a patent ductus arteriosus).

TABLE II—*Sensitivity, specificity, and positive and negative predictive values of clinical examination, chest radiography, electrocardiography, and the three techniques combined*

Diagnostic test	Sensitivity	Specificity	Predictive value: Positive	Predictive value: Negative
Clinical examination	0·53	0·94	0·86	0·73
Chest radiography	0·44	0·98	0·94	0·71
Electrocardiography	0·41	1·0	1·0	0·71
Three techniques combined*	0·71	0·91	0·86	0·81

*At least one technique giving a positive result.

TABLE I—*Positive and negative diagnoses of heart disease in 81 babies with Down's syndrome by clinical examination, chest radiography, electrocardiography, and their combination compared with results of echocardiography. Values are numbers of cases*

	Clinical examination		Chest radiography		Electrocardiography*		Three combined	
	Positive	Negative	Positive	Negative	Positive	Negative	Positive	Negative
Echocardiography:								
Negative	3	44	1	46	0	47	4	43
Positive	18	16	15	19	13	19	24	10

*Not performed in two cases.

Discussion

The incidence of Down's syndrome for the two years of the study was 1·50 per 1000 live births (or one in 670). This is in keeping with that generally quoted with our experience in Northern Ireland: the average annual incidence for 1980-9 was 1·47 per 1000 live births (95% confidence interval 1·38 to 1·56). The incidences of congenital heart disease and of the three major types of cardiac defects were similar to those found by some workers[2,3] but different from those found by others.[4] These differences reflect the nature of previous studies. Few prospective studies of congenital heart disease in

Down's syndrome have been performed[2]; most have been retrospective and some have included only children with known cardiac disease examined at cardiac catheterisation[3,4] or at necropsy.[6,7] We studied all babies with Down's syndrome irrespective of whether they had symptoms or signs. Cross sectional Doppler echocardiography in a logical sequential approach can accurately detect most cardiac defects[8]; to date none of the babies in our study who had echocardiographically normal hearts have been referred back because of cardiac problems. Our results therefore probably reflect the true incidence of congenital heart disease in the population studied.

Screening for congenital heart disease by clinical examination, chest radiography, electrocardiography, or a combination of all three of these techniques may fail to detect clinically important defects in the neonatal period. The sensitivity of each of the techniques alone was low, though it was improved when they were used in combination. This insensitivity might be due because symptoms are not present and clinical and radiological signs of a left to right shunt may not have developed in the immediate postnatal period owing to the high pulmonary vascular resistance at this time.[2] Electrocardiograms may be abnormal, particularly in the presence of an atrioventricular septal defect[2,4]; we found that an abnormal electrocardiogram had a high positive predictive value for congenital heart disease. In some units neonatal electrocardiography may not be readily available or the results incorrectly interpreted because of unfamiliarity with normal findings in the newborn. Diagnosis is rapid, non-invasive, and definitive by echocardiography. It is best performed under the direction of paediatric cardiologists, who have the necessary equipment, technical skill, and clinical experience. The introduction of screening of all babies with Down's syndrome should not result in a major increase in workload for individual paediatric cardiologists; in Northern Ireland this would mean less than one extra new patient a week.

Pulmonary vascular disease is more common and occurs at an earlier stage in babies with Down's syndrome and congenital heart disease,[9] particularly in those with large left to right shunts.[9,10] Such babies have a higher pulmonary artery pressure both at cardiac catheterisation[10] and preoperatively than have normal babies.[11] About 30-40% of children have irreversible changes precluding surgery at the time of presentation.[10,11] Whether these babies should be offered surgery has been a subject of some debate.[12-14] In Northern Ireland the policy is to offer the full range of treatment to such children, unless the treatment is contraindicated or not desired by their parents. In some centres surgery is not routinely offered as the actuarial survival without treatment is thought to be similar to or better than than that of children treated surgically.[12] Recent evidence suggests, however, that the actuarial survival of babies who have had surgery for atrioventricular septal defects is much better than of those treated by medical means alone[15]; most of these babies have Down's syndrome. This is partly related to improvements in surgical skill, though the time of surgical intervention is also critical; operation performed after the first year of life has twice the mortality of surgery before the first year,[11] mainly because pulmonary vascular changes develop after only six months of life in Down's syndrome.[16] In this study we did not determine whether earlier detection and subsequent management of congenital heart disease had any effect on morbidity or outcome. This is an important but peripheral issue that can be investigated only by a randomised controlled trial, if such a trial is ethically justified.

Many parents of babies with Down's syndrome are aware of the increased risk of congenital heart disease and would be reassured by a normal echocardiogram. When it is abnormal parents can be informed at an early stage and counselled appropriately. Early diagnosis of congenital heart disease, particularly of large left to right shunts, could enable a paediatrician to follow the baby carefully, to start medical treatment with diuretics and digoxin at an earlier stage, and possibly to plan for earlier surgical intervention should this be indicated. We believe that babies with Down's syndrome should be screened for congenital heart disease in units where surgery, when needed, is a normal treatment option. Screening should preferably be by echocardiography as this is highly sensitive and specific compared with other methods. Babies should be seen as early in life as possible, preferably in the first six months before pulmonary vascular disease can develop. Surveillance of recent laboratory records by the regional medical genetics service is an important adjunct, permitting the detection of new cases that are not referred by clinicians, and should be included in the screening process when possible.

We thank all the obstetricians and paediatricians who diligently referred their patients to us; the medical genetics laboratory staff and Jayne Rogers for their expert technical help; and Dr Mark Reid for his help and encouragement during this study.

1 Elwood JM, Darragh PM. Severe mental handicap in Northern Ireland. *J Ment Defic Res* 1981;25:147-55.
2 Rowe RD, Uchida IA. Cardiac malformations in mongolism: a prospective study of 184 mongoloid children. *Am J Med* 1961;31:726-35.
3 Cullum L, Liebman J. The association of congenital heart disease with Down's syndrome (Mongolism). *Am J Cardiol* 1969;24:354-7.
4 Shaher RM, Farina MA, Porter IH, Bishop M. Clinical aspects of congenital heart disease in mongolism. *Am J Cardiol* 1972;29:497-503.
5 Ades AE. Evaluating screening tests and screening programmes. *Arch Dis Child* 1990;65:792-5.
6 Tandon R, Edwards JE. Cardiac malformations associated with Down's syndrome. *Circulation* 1973;47:1349-55.
7 Park SC, Matthews RA, Zuberbuhler JR, Rowe RD, Neches WH, Lenox CC. Down syndrome with congenital heart malformation. *Am J Dis Child* 1977;131:29-33.
8 Gussenhoven EJ, Becker AE. Sequential segemental analysis in complex congenital heart disease: an echopathological correlation. In: Marcelleti C, Anderson RH, Becker AE, Corno A, di Carlo D, Mazzera E, eds. *Paediatric cardiology*. Vol 6. Edinburgh: Churchill Livingstone, 1986:156-71.
9 Greenwood RD, Nadas AS. The clinical course of cardiac disease in Down's syndrome. *Pediatrics* 1976;58:893-7.
10 Sondon P, Stijns M, Tremouroux-Wattiej M, Vliers A. Precocity of pulmonary vascular obstruction in Down's syndrome. *European Journal of Cardiology* 1975;2:473-6.
11 Morray JP, MacGillivray R, Duker G. Increased perioperative risk following repair of congenital heart disease in Down's syndrome. *Anesthesiology* 1986;65:221-4.
12 Bull C, Rigby M, Shinebourne EA. Should management of complete atrioventricular canal defect be influenced by coexistant Down syndrome? *Lancet* 1985;i:1147-9.
13 Wilson NJ, Gavalaki E, Newman CGH. Complete atrioventricular septal defect in the presence of Down syndrome. *Lancet* 1985;ii:834.
14 Johnson AM. Management of cardiac disease in Down's syndrome. *Devel Med Child Neurol* 1978;20:220-3.
15 Frontera-Izquerdo P, Cabezuelo-Huerta G. Natural and modified history of complete atrioventricular septal defect—a 17 year study. *Arch Dis Child* 1990;65:964-7.
16 Newfeld EA, Sher M, Paul MH, Nikaidoh H. Pulmonary vascular disease in complete atrioventricular canal. *Am J Cardiol* 1977;39:721-6.

(Accepted 4 April 1991)

DIAGNOSIS WORKSHEET: 1 of 2

Clinical question:

Are the results of this diagnostic study valid?

Was there an independent, blind comparison with a reference ('gold') standard of diagnosis?

Was the diagnostic test evaluated in an appropriate spectrum of patients (like those in whom it would be used in practice)?

Was the reference standard applied regardless of the diagnostic test result?

Are the valid results of this diagnostic study important?

SAMPLE CALCULATIONS (see p 120 in *Evidence-based Medicine*):

		Target disorder (iron deficiency anaemia)		**Totals**
		Present	Absent	
Diagnostic test result (serum ferritin)	Positive (<65 mmol/L)	731 a	270 b	1001 a + b
	Negative (≥65 mmol/L)	78 c	1500 d	1578 c + d
	Totals	809 a + c	1770 b + d	2579 a + b + c + d

Sensitivity = a/(a+c) = 731/809 = 90%

Specificity = d/(b+d) = 1500/1770 = 85%

Likelihood Ratio for a positive test result = LR+ = sens/(1–spec) = 90%/15% = 6

Likelihood Ratio for a negative test result = LR– = (1–sens)/spec = 10%/85% = 0.12

Positive Predictive Value = a/(a+b) = 731/1001 = 73%

Negative Predictive Value = d/(c+d) = 1500/1578 = 95%

Pre-test Probability (prevalence) = (a+c)/(a+b+c+d) = 809/2579 = 32%

Pre-test-odds = prevalence/(1–prevalence) = 31%/69% = 0.45

Post-test odds = Pre-test odds × Likelihood Ratio

Post-test Probability = Post-test odds/(Post-test odds + 1)

YOUR CALCULATIONS

		Target disorder		**Totals**
		Present	Absent	
Diagnostic test result	Positive	a	b	a + b
	Negative	c	d	c + d
	Totals	a + c	b + d	a + b + c + d

Sensitivity = a/(a+c) =

Specificity = d/(b+d) =

Likelihood Ratio for a positive test result = LR+ = sens/(1–spec) =

Likelihood Ratio for a negative test result = LR– = (1–sens)/spec =

Positive Predictive Value = a/(a+b) =

Negative Predictive Value = d/(c+d) =

Pre-test Probability (prevalence) = (a+c)/(a+b+c+d) =

Pre-test-odds = prevalence/(1–prevalence) =

Post-test odds = Pre-test odds × Likelihood Ratio =

Post-test Probability = Post-test odds/(Post-test odds + 1) =

Can you apply this valid, important evidence about a diagnostic test in caring for your patient?	
Is the diagnostic test available, affordable, accurate, and precise in your setting?	
Can you generate a clinically sensible estimate of your patient's pre-test probability (from practice data, from personal experience, from the report itself, or from clinical speculation)	
Will the resulting post-test probabilities affect your management and help your patient? (Could it move you across a test-treatment threshold? Would your patient be a willing partner in carrying it out?)	
Would the consequences of the test help your patient?	

Additional notes

A LIKELIHOOD RATIO NOMOGRAM

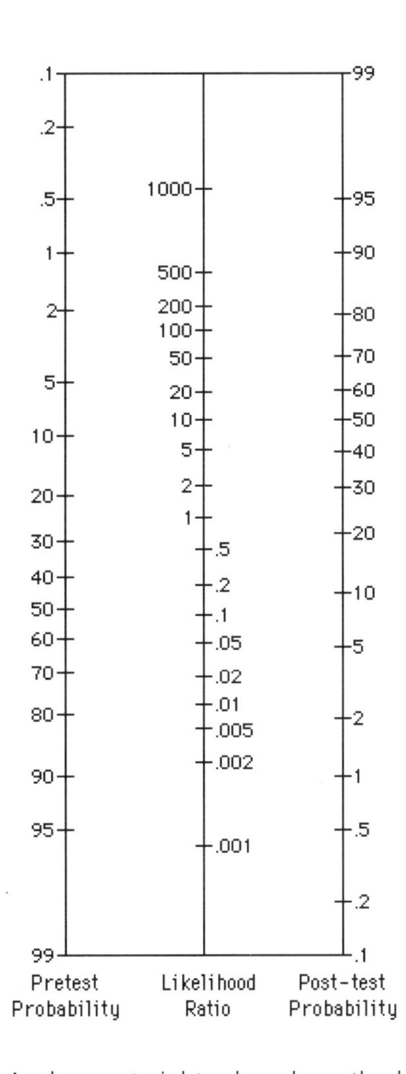

Anchor a straight edge along the left edge of the nomogram at your patient's pre-test probability and pivot it until it intersects the likelihood ratio for your patient's diagnostic test result. It will intersect the right edge of the nomogram at your patient's post-test probability. Test 1: for a likelihood ratio of 1, pre-test and post-test probabilities should be identical. Test 2: for a pre-test probability of 30% and a likelihood ratio of 5, the post-test probability is just under 70%.

Adapted from Fagan TJ (1975) Nomogram for Bayes' theorem. *NEJM* **293:** 257.

COMPLETED DIAGNOSIS WORKSHEET: 1 of 2

Clinical question: In babies affected by Down's syndrome, how useful are clinical examination, CXR and ECG in predicting the risk of congenital heart disease?

Are the results of this diagnostic study valid?

Was there an independent, blind comparison with a reference ('gold') standard of diagnosis?	**Yes. All examined by cardiac ECHO. Person doing ECHO was probably not blind to other examination results.**
Was the diagnostic test evaluated in an appropriate spectrum of patients (like those in whom it would be used in practice)?	**Yes. All babies with Down's syndrome in the region. Unlikely that any cases missed.**
Was the reference standard applied regardless of the diagnostic test result?	**Yes, eventually, most during early infancy.**

Are the valid results of this diagnostic study important?

YOUR CALCULATIONS

		Heart disease (ECHO)		Totals
		Present	**Absent**	
Diagnostic test result (clinical examination)	Positive	18 a	3 b	21 a + b
	Negative	16 c	44 d	60 c + d
	Totals	34 a + c	47 b + d	81 a + b + c + d

Sensitivity = a/(a+c) = **52.9%**

Specificity = d/(b+d) = **93.6%**

Likelihood Ratio for a positive test result = LR+ = sens/(1–spec) **= 8.3**

Likelihood Ratio for a negative test result=LR– = (1–sens)/spec **= 0.5**

Positive Predictive Value = a/(a+b) = **86%**

Negative Predictive Value = d/(c+d) = **73%**

Pre-test Probability (prevalence) = (a+c)/(a+b+c+d) = **42%**

Pre-test-odds = prevalence/(1–prevalence) = **0.72**

Post-test odds for negative test result = Pre-test odds × Likelihood Ratio = **0.72** × **0.5 = 0.36**

Post-test Probability for negative test result = Post-test odds/(Post-test odds + 1) = **26%**

COMPLETED DIAGNOSIS WORKSHEET: 2 of 2

Can you apply this valid, important evidence about a diagnostic test in caring for your patient?	
Is the diagnostic test available, affordable, accurate, and precise in your setting?	**Yes.**
Can you generate a clinically sensible estimate of your patient's pre-test probability (from practice data, from personal experience, from the report itself, or from clinical speculation)	**Yes. Unlikely to differ from that used in the study.**
Will the resulting post-test probabilities affect your management and help your patient? (Could it move you across a test-treatment threshold? Would your patient be a willing partner in carrying it out?)	**Depends on results. Negative tests don't move patient across management threshold (i.e. would still want ECHO). If use 26% (after exam) as new pre-test probability, post-test probability after normal CXR will be 17% (LR for –ve CXR = 0.57). 17% chance of congenital heart disease still high.**
Would the consequences of the test help your patient?	**Yes. A positive examination is helpful. A negative examination still requires ECHO. Very little additional information provided by chest X-ray or ECG if examination is negative.**

Additional notes

1 It is important that the 2 × 2 table is the correct orientation (i.e. gold standard on the top). Note that Table 1 on page 1426 needs to be re-oriented.
2 ECG : is a SpPin (Specificity = 100% and positive ECG rules in diagnosis).
3 Can use post-test probability of one test as pre-test probability of the next test (as long as the tests are independent). It is unlikely the clinical examination and chest X-ray are truly independent, which over-estimates the likelihood ratio.
4 Emphasise the importance of thinking about the confidence intervals around likelihood ratios.

A LIKELIHOOD RATIO NOMOGRAM

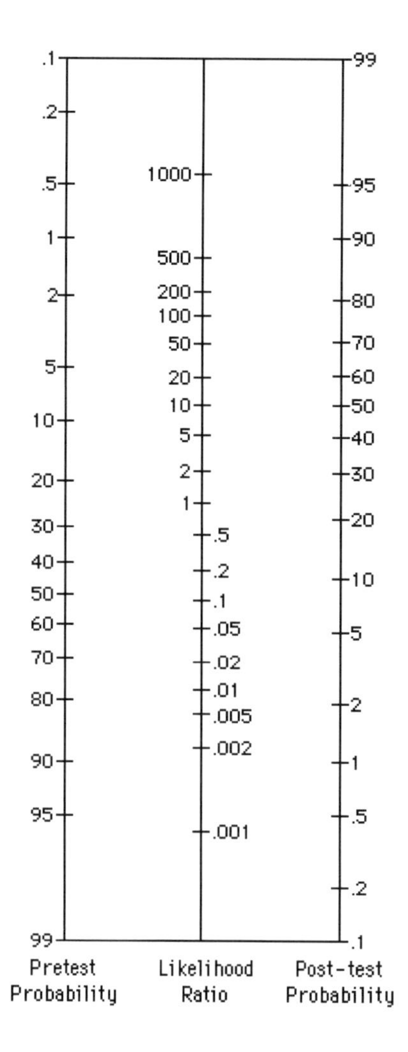

Anchor a straight edge along the left edge of the nomogram at your patient's pre-test probability and pivot it until it intersects the likelihood ratio for your patient's diagnostic test result. It will intersect the right edge of the nomogram at your patient's post-test probability. Test 1: for a likelihood ratio of 1, pre-test and post-test probabilities should be identical. Test 2: for a pre-test probability of 30% and a likelihood ratio of 5, the post-test probability is just under 70%.

Adapted from Fagan TJ (1975) Nomogram for Bayes' theorem. *NEJM* **293:** 257.

DOWN'S SYNDROME – NORMAL CLINICAL EXAM, CXR AND ECG DON'T RULE OUT CONGENITAL HEART DISEASE

Appraised by O Duperrex and R Gilbert: 14 May 1999
Expiry date: March 2000.

Clinical Bottom Line

Clinical examination should be followed by echocardiography to detect congenital heart disease in babies affected by Down's syndrome. Babies with a normal clinical examination, chest X-ray and ECG still have a 19% risk of congenital heart disease.

Citation

Tubman TRJ, Shields MD, Craig BG, Mulholland HC and Nevin NC (1991) Congenital heart disease in Down's Syndrome: two year prospective early screening study. *BMJ* **302:** 1425–7.

Clinical Question

In babies affected by Down's syndrome, how useful are clinical examination, chest X-ray or ECG in predicting their risk of congenital heart disease?

Search Terms

'Down's-Syndrome' and 'newborn' and 'clinical examination' and 'X-Ray' and ('diagnosis' or 'sensitivity-and-specificity').

The Study

1 Reference standard – echocardiography (cross-sectional Doppler) applied to all patients.
2 Test – clinical examination (cyanosis, tachypnoea, abnormal precordial impulse or murmur), ECG (QRS axis abnormal or evidence of LVH), chest X-ray (CXR, as reported by radiologist).
3 Study setting – ascertainment of all infants affected by Down's syndrome in the region through notification by paediatricians and obstetricians, regional cytogenetics services, and regional paediatric cardiology service (Northern Ireland, 1987–89).

The Evidence

Test	LR+ (95%CI)	LR– (95%CI)
Clinical examination	8.3 (2.7–26)	0.50 (0.35–0.72)
Chest X-ray	21 (2.9–150)	0.57 (0.42–0.77)
ECG	Infinity	0.59 (0.45–0.79)
Three combined*	8.3 (3.2–22)	0.32 (0.19–0.55)

*Any 1/3 pos is considered as pos; all neg is considered as neg

Baseline risk of congenital heart disease was 42% (34/81).

If all tests are negative, risk of congenital heart disease = 19%

Comments

1 ECHO is unlikely to have been performed blind to the other test results.
2 In newborns affected by Down's syndrome, a positive examination, chest X-ray or ECG strongly predict congenital heart disease.
3 A negative examination, chest X-ray and/or ECG is not clinically useful.

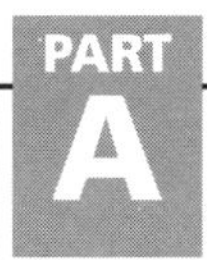

EBCH SESSION

2

SECTION 2

Diagnosis and asking answerable clinical questions

PART A Critical appraisal of a clinical article about diagnosis

Section 2: Ultrasound for pyloric stenosis

A 5-week-old baby boy has been admitted with projectile vomiting. You are unable to palpate a pyloric tumour. You decide to admit the child and observe him at least for the next 24 hours. However, the parents are keen to take their child home now.

You ask for an ultrasound of the pylorus and the radiologist reports the result as negative. Do you send the child home? You pose the question, in young infants with projectile vomiting and no palpable pyloric tumour, what is the probability of pyloric stenosis with a negative or a positive ultrasound of the pylorus?

You search Medline using the terms 'pyloric stenosis' and 'ultrasound' and find the following paper. Neilson D, Hollman AS (1994) The ultrasonic diagnosis of infantile hypertrophic pyloric stenosis:technique and accuracy. *Clinical Radiology* **49:** 246–7.

Read the following article and decide:

1 Are the results of this diagnostic article valid?
2 Are the valid results of this diagnostic study important?
3 Can you apply this valid, important evidence about a diagnostic test in caring for your patient?

If you want to read some strategies for answering these sorts of questions, you could have a look at pp 81–4, 118–28 and 159–63 in *Evidence-based Medicine*.

PART B Asking answerable clinical questions

We will illustrate the importance, strategies, and tactics of formulating clinical questions and work with you on the 3–4 parts of the question.

Participants will break up into groups of two, discuss patients they cared for in the previous week, and generate questions they think are important concerning their patients' therapy, diagnosis and prognosis.

In larger groups, we will review and refine the questions, and then keep track of them as possible questions to use in later sessions devoted to searching for the best evidence.

Clinical Radiology (1994) 49, 246–247

The Ultrasonic Diagnosis of Infantile Hypertrophic Pyloric Stenosis: Technique and Accuracy

D. NEILSON and A. S. HOLLMAN

Department of Radiology, The Royal Hospital for Sick Children, Glasgow

The role of ultrasound for the diagnosis of pyloric stenosis has yet to be definitely established. We have carried out 147 ultrasound examinations of 142 infants (99 male and 43 female) with a history of projectile vomiting or the possibility of a pyloric mass. Measurements of the pyloric canal length, transverse pyloric diameter and muscle wall thickness were taken from a longitudinal view of the pylorus and related to previously described control data. The accuracy of the ultrasound examination was related to the finally established diagnosis. The results obtained revealed a sensitivity of 97% and specificity of 99% with positive predictive value of 99%. The three diagnostic errors (1 false positive and 2 false negative) occurred during the 'learning curve' of the radiologists and were the *15th, 29th* and *35th* cases examined, indicating that almost a 100% accuracy can potentially be achieved. This study confirms that ultrasound examination is the first line of investigation in a child in whom the clinical diagnosis of hypertrophic pyloric stenosis is uncertain and indicates that unnecessary surgery can thereby be prevented. Neilson, D. & Hollman, A.S. (1994). *Clinical Radiology* 49, 246–247. The Ultrasonic Diagnosis of Infantile Hypertrophic Pyloric Stenosis: Technique and Accuracy

Accepted for Publication 14 September 1993

Ultrasound assessment of the pylorus has been reported to have an accuracy of between 81% [1] and 100% [2] for the diagnosis of infantile hypertrophic pyloric stenosis (HPS). Clinical assessment alone can be accurate in up to 90% of cases, in which a small test feed is administered, and a pyloric tumour palpated. However, considerable clinical skill and, on occasion, multiple examinations are required to identify the hypertrophied pylorus, hence radiological evaluation is commonly requested for infants with projectile vomiting but no palpable mass.

Although pyloric ultrasound is now a well established technique [3], a recent article from Australia casts doubt on the value of radiological imaging and suggests that surgery may well be delayed by waiting for ultrasound [4]. Another article has suggested 'it remains to be seen whether ultrasound will prove accurate when the clinical diagnosis is in doubt' [5], and other authors [6] have suggested that 'its use for diagnosis seems doubtful'. These authors advocate confirmation of the diagnosis by a barium meal.

The ultrasonic method and expertise used to assess the pylorus, and the interpretation of the results obtained, clearly determine the ultimate sensitivity and specificity of the investigation. We report the details of the technique used in the Royal Hospital for Sick Children, Glasgow, and the outcome of a retrospective audit of our results.

PATIENTS AND METHODS

Over a three and a half year period, 142 infants (99 males and 43 females) under the age of 5 months were referred for pyloric ultrasound. All infants were examined clinically by senior paediatric surgical staff, and radiologically by consultant paediatric radiologists. All babies had a history of projectile vomiting in whom a pyloric tumour had not been palpated, or where there was some controversy at different test feed examinations about the presence of a pyloric mass. The accuracy of the ultrasonic examinations were then correlated with a review of the final diagnosis and operative findings for all cases.

The ultrasound examination technique is as described by Stunden *et al.* [2]. A nasogastric tube was inserted on the ward by the nursing staff beforehand, and in the ultrasonic department the milk curd residue is aspirated and replaced by 30–40 ml of sterile water. This is repeated until aspirate is clear. Gastric filling is titrated using ultrasound to ensure an over distended stomach is avoided. The water provides a clear echo-free landmark and window through which to visualize the pylorus, found in a very constant position adjacent or behind the water-filled gastric antrum. The infant is examined lying on their right side in a semi-erect position using a 7MHz sector scanner (Acuson 128XP). Measurements are taken of the pyloric canal length, transverse pyloric diameter and muscle wall thickness from a longitudinal view of the pylorus. This is usually achieved by scanning the abdomen transversely. An irritable infant can be quietened using a dummy with a small amount of glycerine on it.

The criteria for confirming a diagnosis of pyloric stenosis were those of Stunden *et al.* [2] indicated in Table 1. If a positive diagnosis was made the nasogastric tube was left *in situ* until surgery. The tube is removed if a negative diagnosis was made.

RESULTS

One hundred and forty-seven ultrasound examinations were performed on 142 infants. Two babies had two scans each, and one infant had four ultrasonic examinations as he was managed with conservative treatment, after parental refusal for surgical intervention.

Correspondence to: Dr A. S. Hollman, Department of Radiology, The Royal Hospital for Sick Children, Yorkhill, Glasgow G3 8SJ.

Table 1 – Features of the normal and abnormal pylorus

	Normal	*Abnormal*
Canal length	Less than 15 mm	Greater than 16 mm
Transverse pyloric diameter	Usually 11 mm or less	Usually over 11 mm
Muscle wall thickness	Less than 2.5 mm thick	More than 2.5 mm thick
Relaxation of pylorus	Pylorus relaxes	Canal does not open
Gastric peristalsis	Normal	Increased
Passage of gastric water feed	Normal gastric emptying	Little passage of contents

Table 2 – Accuracy of ultrasound diagnosis in 147 examinations in 142 infants

True positive	66	Sensitivity 97%
True negative	78	Specificity 99%
False positive	1	Positive predictive value 99%
False negative	2	
Total	147	

Sixty-seven examinations were positive (Table 2) in whom 66 of these infants had a diagnosis of pyloric stenosis confirmed at surgery. A false positive diagnosis was made on an 8-week-old infant recovering from necrotizing enterocolitis. An initial examination was reported as normal, but a subsequent one 3 weeks later was reported to show pyloric hypertrophy and was incorrectly diagnosed as pyloric stenosis, although water was noted to empty through the pylorus throughout the examination. At operation the baby was found to have non-obstructive pyloric hypertrophy.

There were 78 true negative examinations and two false negative scans. The first false negative examination was reported as showing pyloric hypertrophy (but not stenosis) in a 2-week-old infant. A repeat follow-up examination was offered but with continued vomiting pyloric stenosis was found at operation 3 days later. The other showed 'gastric outlet obstruction, pylorus not identified'. On the strength of this, an operation was performed confirming pyloric stenosis.

These results give a sensitivity of 97% and a specificity of 99%, with predictive value of a positive test of 99%.

DISCUSSION

Ultrasonic diagnosis of hypertrophic pyloric stenosis in infants was first reported in 1977 by Teele and Smith [7]. Since then various techniques have been described of how to scan the pylorus of babies presenting with projectile vomiting and the accuracy of these techniques has varied widely.

The technique described by Stunden *et al.* [2] is simple and allows rapid diagnosis, earlier operation and discharge. The use of the nasogastric tube has several advantages over an oral water feed. The highly echogenic milk curds can be removed from the stomach, and the water instilled provides a clear acoustic window to visualize the pylorus. The tube removes the need for fasting the baby before the scan, and also removes the need for patient co-operation. We have found many infants are reluctant to bottle feed from sterile water or % dextrose, particularly if breast fed. This technique also ensures the infant is much less likely to vomit or aspirate, as gastric distention can be controlled.

The one false positive examination was an infant incorrectly diagnosed as having pyloric stenosis due to operator inexperience. The baby had definite pyloric hypertrophy but the pyloric canal was noted to open widely during the procedure. This condition of non-obstructive pyloric hypertrophy is well recognized [2].

Some controversy remains about which diagnostic criteria should be applied to confirm a positive diagnosis of pyloric stenosis. We have used the criteria [2] of a pyloric canal length $\geqslant 16$ mm, diameter of the pylorus $\geqslant 11$ mm, and muscle thickness $\geqslant 2.5$ mm as abnormal, with emphasis on the dynamic appearance of the pylorus in observing whether the pylorus opens widely or not during the feed. We have achieved a sensitivity of 97%, specificity of 99% and positive predictive value of 99%, confirming the validity of these criteria. We have found very few examinations in which these criteria have been difficult to apply or in which the measurements are borderline and the examination is non-diagnostic.

In our practice, pyloric ultrasound is a freely available service, usually performed within a couple of hours of presentation. The 66 true positive examinations represent 23% of the total number of cases eventually having a pyloromyotomy during the study period. This is within the accepted range of 'clinically difficult' cases of HPS that would otherwise require repeated test feeds or a barium meal, and suggests that the ultrasound service is being used appropriately as a rapid, safe adjunct to clinical examination, not a substitute.

Acknowledgements. We would like to thank all our surgical colleagues for referring the infants and to Dr M. A. Ziervogel who performed some of the studies.

REFERENCES

1 Pilling DW. Infantile hypertrophic pyloric stenosis: a fresh approach to diagnosis. *Clinical Radiology* 1983;34(1):51–53.
2 Stunden RJ, LeQuesne GW, Little KET. The improved ultrasound diagnosis of hypertrophic pyloric stenosis. *Paediatric Radiology* 1986;16:200–205.
3 Carver RA, Okorie M, Steiner GM, Dickson JND. Infantile hypertrophic pyloric stenosis – diagnosis from the pyloric muscle index. *Clinical Radiology* 1987;38:625–627.
4 Macdessi J, Oates RK. Clinical diagnosis of pyloric stenosis: a declining art. *British Medical Journal* 1993;306:553–555.
5 Kiely EM. Commentary. *Archives of Diseases of Childhood* 1991;66:132–133.
6 Eriksen CA, Anders CJ. Audit of results of operations for infantile pyloric stenosis in a district general hospital. *Archives of Diseases of Childhood* 1991;66:130–132.
7 Teele RL, Smith EH. Ultrasound in the diagnosis of idiopathic hypertrophic pyloric stenosis. *New England Journal of Medicine* 1977;296:1149–1150.

DIAGNOSIS WORKSHEET: 1 of 2

Clinical question:

Are the results of this diagnostic study valid?

Was there an independent, blind comparison with a reference ('gold') standard of diagnosis?

Was the diagnostic test evaluated in an appropriate spectrum of patients (like those in whom it would be used in practice)?

Was the reference standard applied regardless of the diagnostic test result?

Are the valid results of this diagnostic study important?

SAMPLE CALCULATIONS (*see* p 120 *Evidence-based Medicine*):

		Target disorder (iron deficiency anaemia)		**Totals**
		Present	Absent	
Diagnostic test result (serum ferritin)	Positive (<65 mmol/L)	731 a	270 b	1001 a + b
	Negative (≥65 mmol/L)	78 c	1500 d	1578 c + d
	Totals	809 a + c	1770 b + d	2579 a + b + c + d

Sensitivity = a/(a+c) = 731/809 = 90%

Specificity = d/(b+d) = 1500/1770 = 85%

Likelihood Ratio for a positive test result = LR+ = sens/(1–spec) = 90%/15% = 6

Likelihood Ratio for a negative test result = LR– = (1–sens)/spec =10%/85% = 0.12

Positive Predictive Value = a/(a+b) = 731/1001 = 73%

Negative Predictive Value = d/(c+d) = 1500/1578 = 95%

Pre-test Probability (prevalence) = (a+c)/(a+b+c+d) = 809/2579 = 32%

Pre-test-odds = prevalence/(1–prevalence) = 31%/69% = 0.45

Post-test odds = Pre-test odds × Likelihood Ratio

Post-test Probability = Post-test odds/(Post-test odds + 1)

YOUR CALCULATIONS

		Target disorder		Totals
		Present	Absent	
Diagnostic test result	Positive	a	b	a + b
	Negative	c	d	c + d
	Totals	a + c	b + d	a + b + c + d

Sensitivity = a/(a+c) =

Specificity = d/(b+d) =

Likelihood Ratio for a positive test result = LR+ = sens/(1–spec) =

Likelihood Ratio for a negative test result = LR– = (1–sens)/spec =

Positive Predictive Value = a/(a+b) =

Negative Predictive Value = d/(c+d) =

Pre-test Probability (prevalence) = (a+c)/(a+b+c+d) =

Pre-test-odds = prevalence/(1–prevalence) =

Post-test odds = Pre-test odds × Likelihood Ratio =

Post-test Probability = Post-test odds/(Post-test odds + 1) =

Can you apply this valid, important evidence about a diagnostic test in caring for your patient?

Is the diagnostic test available, affordable, accurate, and precise in your setting?	
Can you generate a clinically sensible estimate of your patient's pre-test probability (from practice data, from personal experience, from the report itself, or from clinical speculation)	
Will the resulting post-test probabilities affect your management and help your patient? (Could it move you across a test-treatment threshold? Would your patient be a willing partner in carrying it out?)	
Would the consequences of the test help your patient?	

Additional notes

A LIKELIHOOD RATIO NOMOGRAM

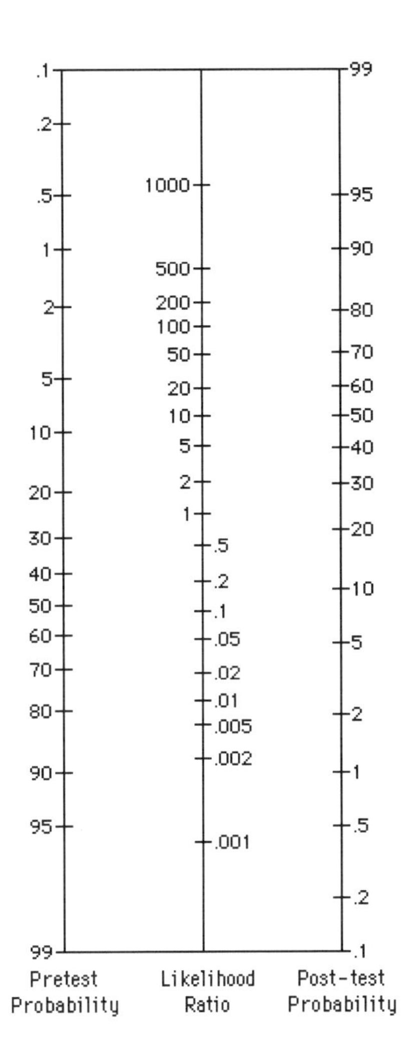

Anchor a straight edge along the left edge of the nomogram at your patient's pre-test probability and pivot it until it intersects the likelihood ratio for your patient's diagnostic test result. It will intersect the right edge of the nomogram at your patient's post-test probability. Test 1: for a likelihood ratio of 1, pre-test and post-test probabilities should be identical. Test 2: for a pre-test probability of 30% and a likelihood ratio of 5, the post-test probability is just under 70%.

Adapted from Fagan TJ (1975) Nomogram for Bayes' theorem. *NEJM* **293:** 257.

COMPLETED DIAGNOSIS WORKSHEET: 1 of 2

Clinical question: In infants with projectile vomiting in whom there is no palpable tumour, does ultrasound aid in diagnosis (rule in or out) of pyloric stenosis?

Are the results of this diagnostic study valid?

Was there an independent, blind comparison with a reference ('gold') standard of diagnosis?	**Yes. All followed until hospital discharge. Length of follow up not given.**
Was the diagnostic test evaluated in an appropriate spectrum of patients (like those in whom it would be used in practice)?	**Yes. In infants with an equivocal diagnosis.**
Was the reference standard applied regardless of the diagnostic test result?	**Yes. All followed up until discharge. We assume that pyloric stenosis will not resolve spontaneously; this may not be true.**

Are the valid results of this diagnostic study important?

YOUR CALCULATIONS

		Pyloric stenosis		**Totals**
		Present	**Absent**	
Diagnostic test result (USS)	Positive	66 a	1 b	67 a + b
	Negative	2 c	78 d	80 c + d
	Totals	68 a + c	79 b + d	147 a + b + c + d

Sensitivity = a/(a+c) = 97.1%

Specificity = d/(b+d) = 98.7%

Likelihood Ratio for a positive test result = LR+ = sens/(1–spec) = 75

Likelihood Ratio for a negative test result = LR– = (1–sens)/spec = 0.03

Positive Predictive Value = a/(a+b) = 99%

Negative Predictive Value = d/(c+d) = 98%

Pre-test Probability (prevalence) = (a+c)/(a+b+c+d) = 46%

Pre-test-odds = prevalence/(1–prevalence) = 0.85

Post-test odds for a negative result = Pre-test odds × Likelihood Ratio = 0.85 × 0.03 = 0.0255

Post-test Probability for a negative result = Post-test odds/(Post-test odds + 1) = 2.5%

COMPLETED DIAGNOSIS WORKSHEET: 2 of 2

Can you apply this valid, important evidence about a diagnostic test in caring for your patient?	
Is the diagnostic test available, affordable, accurate, and precise in your setting?	**Yes.**
Can you generate a clinically sensible estimate of your patient's pre-test probability (from practice data, from personal experience, from the report itself, or from clinical speculation)	**Yes. Could audit own practice if don't feel 46% of babies with projectile vomiting and no tumour palpable is realistic.**
Will the resulting post-test probabilities affect your management and help your patient? (Could it move you across a test-treatment threshold? Would your patient be a willing partner in carrying it out?)	**Depends on results. Negative test means post-test probability now <5%, and you would be happy for baby to go home. Both +ve and –ve tests move patient across treatment thresholds.**
Would the consequences of the test help your patient?	**Yes. Earlier discharge if negative. Earlier surgery if positive.**

Additional notes

1. This is a SpPin (Specificity = 99% so positive ultrasound scan (USS) rules in diagnosis).
2. In fact, there were only 142 patients and 5 of USS were reexaminations. Only first USS should have been included in results. It is apparent that repeat scans were performed mostly on true positive or true negative cases, which means sensitivity and specificity will not be altered greatly.
3. If the surgeon knew the result of the USS (i.e. not blind), this might exaggerate sensitivity and specificity.
4. Emphasise the importance of thinking about the confidence intervals around the likelihood ratios (CATMaker generates these for you).

A LIKELIHOOD RATIO NOMOGRAM

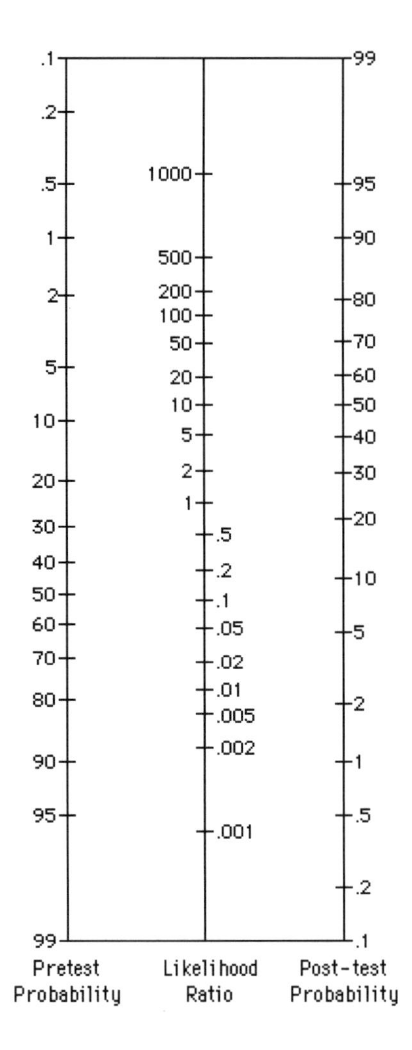

Anchor a straight edge along the left edge of the nomogram at your patient's pre-test probability and pivot it until it intersects the likelihood ratio for your patent's diagnostic test result. It will intersect the right edge of the nomogram at your patient's post-test probability. Test 1: for a likelihood ratio of 1, pre-test and post-test probabilities should be identical. Test 2: for a pre-test probability of 30% and a likelihood ratio of 5, the post-test probability is just under 70%.

Adapted from Fagan TJ (1975) Nomogram for Bayes' theorem. *NEJM* **293:** 257.

PYLORIC STENOSIS – ULTRASOUND IS DIAGNOSTIC

Appraised by O Duperrex and R Gilbert: 14 May 1999
Expiry date: March 2000.

Clinical Bottom Line

In young infants with projective vomiting but no palpable pyloric tumour, ultrasound is useful to rule in and rule out pyloric stenosis.

Citation

Neilson D and Hollman AS (1994) The ultrasonic diagnosis of infantile hypertrophic pyloric stenosis: technique and accuracy. *Clinical Radiology* **49:** 246–7.

Clinical Question

In young infants with projectile vomiting and no palpable pyloric tumour, what is the probability of hypertrophic pyloric stenosis with a negative or a positive ultrasound of the pylorus?

Search Terms

'pyloric-stenosis' and 'infant' and 'ultrasound' and ('diagnosis' or 'sensitivity-and-specificity').

The Study

1 Reference standard – review of final diagnosis (time after test not stated) and operative findings applied to all.
2 Test – ultrasound scan (USS) of the pylorus: considered positive if pyloric canal length ≥ 16 mm, diameter of pylorus ≥ 11 mm, muscle thickness ≥ 2.5 mm and/or dynamic appearance of pylorus.
3 Study setting – retrospective audit of infants less than 5 months old who had projectile vomiting, no clearly palpable pyloric tumour and who were referred for ultrasound.

The Evidence

		Reference standard Pyloric stenosis at follow-up					**95% confidence interval**
		+	–				
Test	+	66	1	67			
USS	–	2	78	80	**LR+**	77	11 to 538
		68	79	147	**LR–**	0.03	0.01 to 0.12
		Pre-test probability				46%	38% to 54%
		Post-test probability			**Test+**	99%	87% to 100%
		Post-test probability			**Test–**	2.5%	0% to 12%

Comments

1 Surgeons deciding diagnosis were not blind to the ultrasound result.
2 Unclear whether positive test result based on one or all of above criteria.
3 Test was always performed by consultant paediatric radiologists.

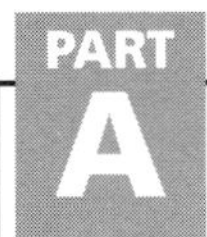

Critical appraisal of a clinical article about prognosis

You are a health visitor doing a Child Health Clinic and are approached by the mother of a 2-year-old boy who has glue ear, manifest by intermittent ear discharge and hearing difficulty. The mother has seen the ENT surgeon who decided against surgery. She wants to know whether glue ear might cause learning and behaviour problems later in childhood. Together you pose the question, will children with middle ear disease have behaviour problems later in childhood?

What do you tell her?

If there is a risk of behaviour problems, she asks whether you think she should pay for private grommet surgery. What is your advice?

You do a Medline search using the terms 'middle ear disease' and 'behaviour problems' and find the enclosed article (*Arch Dis Child* 1999; **80:** 28–35).

Read the article and decide:

1. Is this evidence about prognosis valid?
2. Is the valid evidence about prognosis important?
3. Can you apply this valid and important evidence about prognosis in caring for your patient?
4. If you want to read some strategies for answering these sorts of questions, you could have a look at pp 85–90, 129–32 and 164–5 in *Evidence-based Medicine*, and/or read 'Prognosis – an introduction'.

EBCH SESSION

3

Prognosis and searching the evidence-based journals

PART B

Searching the evidence-based journals

We show you how to search the electronic version of two journals: *ACP Journal Club* (ACPJC) and *Evidence-based Medicine*. The contents of these journals are available on disk as *Best Evidence*. This requires a computer with a CD slot and can be ordered from the BMJ Publishing Group, PO Box 295, London WC1H 9TE; Tel: 0171 387 4499 (subscriptions); Fax: 0171 383 6662; email: bmjsubs@dial.pipex.com

Now would be a good time to start searching on potential topics for your presentations in Sessions 6 and 7!

Behaviour and cognitive outcomes from middle ear disease

Kathleen E Bennett, Mark P Haggard

Abstract
Objectives—To resolve controversies over associations between a history of middle ear disease and psychosocial or cognitive/educational outcomes
Design—Multipurpose longitudinal birth cohort study. Original cohort comprised all UK births between 5 and 11 April 1970; data were available for approximately 12 000 children at 5 years old and 9000 children at 10 years old.
Methods—For 5 year old children, parent reported data were available on health, social, and behavioural factors, including data on two validated markers of middle ear disease. Cognitive tests were administered at 5 and 10 years of age, and behavioural problems rated at 10 years by the child's teacher.
Results—After adjustment for social background and maternal malaise, the developmental sequelae of middle ear disease remained significant even at 10 years. The largest effects were observed in behaviour problems and language test data at age 5, but effect sizes were modest overall.
Implications—These results provide an epidemiological basis for policies that aim to minimise the sequelae of middle ear disease by awareness in parents and preschool teachers, early referral, and intervention for more serious or persistent cases.
(*Arch Dis Child* 1999;80:28–35)

Keywords: middle ear disease; behaviour problems; cognitive development; longitudinal study

MRC Institute of Hearing Research, University Park, Nottingham NG7 2RD, UK
K E Bennett
M P Haggard

Correspondence to: Dr K E Bennett.

Accepted 18 August 1998

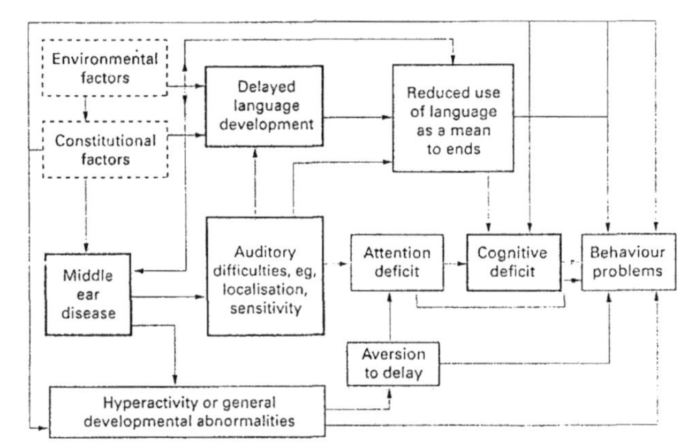

Figure 1 Schema illustrating some possible relations between middle ear disease, illness, hearing, communication, and developmental sequelae.

Otitis media with effusion (OME) or "glue ear" is the most common cause of hearing loss in children; this fluctuating condition can persist in some children, leading to detrimental effects on behaviour and development. Antisocial behaviour or inattentiveness are consequent on the child's inability to hear, leading to frustration, apparent disobedience, and less use of language as a means to ends. Deficits in speech, language, and behaviour, particularly in children with early onset OME, may lead to reduced cognitive ability.[1]

The balance of existing evidence suggests that in most affected children the developmental and behavioural sequelae of otitis media are short lived and relatively mild.[2] Psychosocial and educational outcomes have received less attention than measures of language. Clinical and epidemiological studies suggest some association, but the effect appears small, and the variability wide, probably because of confounding factors that differ between various small samples.[3]

There are advantages in using large longitudinal cohorts to document developmental influences, particularly where these are likely to be complex or to change over time. The prospective stratification (that is, on the middle ear disease variable) which cohort studies permit, greatly reduces the major selection biases present in clinically based studies, such as comorbidity or the tendency to seek care, which may exaggerate the true effects. Most otitis media sequelae studies have lacked sufficient numbers and their designs have not permitted control for factors such as socioeconomic status and maternal depression (or malaise), which are known to be associated with behavioural development or delayed cognition in children.[4] Studies need to take into account the complex set of developmental influences suggested in fig 1.

We have analysed the 1970 British birth cohort (BCS70), a multipurpose longitudinal study, designed to investigate educational, physical, and social development.[5] It is about 10 times larger than any of the other cohorts from Dunedin,[6] Nijmegen,[7] and Boston[8] that have considered behavioural and developmental sequelae of OME. Although these cohort studies provide some of the best evidence of OME sequelae, the numbers of affected children in the Nijmegen and Dunedin studies were small, and the Boston study excluded non-white children and underestimated the occurrence of OME in the children who were tested less frequently.

In our analyses, we emphasise the data on 10 year behaviour assessments, to provide statistical evidence for the more contentious longer term effects of middle ear disease.

Methods

GENERAL METHODOLOGICAL CONSIDERATIONS

Limitations of cohort data

In BCS70, the available markers of the independent variable of middle ear disease are relatively crude: parental reports of suspected/confirmed hearing problems and purulent (non-wax) ear discharge. However, objective measurements repeated over a long period are very expensive, making infeasible any study combining objective markers and the large sample size required for generality, statistical control, and tests of interaction. The total cumulative histories of middle ear disease during childhood, rather than the condition of an ear on a particular day, are what determine sequelae, and are relevant—for example, in deciding whether a child with persistent problems would warrant surgical intervention.

The index group definition is likely to give a conservative estimate of actual disease because the control group will contain some affected children with mild/short term conditions underreported by parents.[9]

Control for confounders

Some of the inherent biases in report can be controlled out. For behavioural and cognitive signs (as distinct from evident problems and symptoms), parental report is likely to be undersensitive. A parent of more advantaged socioeconomic status will be particularly aware and therefore report more hearing problems, but might also have a child with better, not worse, scores on a language scale. This will make the analysis of associations conservative with respect to type I errors on performance measures. For power this is offset by the large number of children for whom complete data are available for analysis. Previous univariate analyses of the 1970 birth cohort[5] have shown that boys are more likely than girls to have reported problems of ear discharge and hearing and, that boys more often exhibit behaviour problems than girls. Our analyses are therefore adjusted for sex as well as socioeconomic status.

SUBJECTS

The original cohort consisted of all births in the UK between 5 and 11 April 1970, with available data on > 12 000 children and additional sweeps at 5, 10, 16, and 21 years.[5] For the analyses that follow, complete data were available on ~ 12 000 children at 5 years of age and ~ 9000 children at 10 years. Owing to mobility, not all the children were traceable, although this did not significantly affect the proportions that had middle ear disease.

INDEPENDENT VARIABLES

At age 5, markers of middle ear disease were reported by parents, in the form of whether or not the child had "suspected hearing difficulty" or "purulent (non-wax) ear discharge" up to the age of 4 as well as between ages 4 and 5. There was little difference in rates of ear problems between these periods, so the data were combined to derive categories "ever" or "never" for each of the reported ear/hearing problem variables up to age 5.

For our analyses, independent variables were the reported ear discharge or hearing difficulty; covariates were maternal malaise, sex, and socioeconomic status. These were the most relevant, although not the only covariates that could have been considered—for example, in this analysis we have not controlled for the child's general health. The socioeconomic status item is a seven value variable (also known as the social index,[10] representing advantaged and disadvantaged children at the extremes) based on a combination of eight items, including fathers' occupation, highest known qualification of either parent, type of accommodation, and neighbourhood. For simplicity of representation, a three valued variable is used grouping the levels of the original seven point social index (one and two; three, four, and five; six and seven).

A maternal malaise score at 5 and 10 years of age was calculated from the sum of items in a 24 item malaise inventory completed by the mother of the cohort member, including items on depression, neuroticism, and feeling miserable. This scale was found previously to discriminate well between those with and without psychiatric disorder.[11]

BEHAVIOUR PROBLEMS

At 5 and 10 years of age, maternally reported behaviour problem data were collected using Rutter A rating scales[11]; at 10 years of age, teacher reported behaviour was collected using a 52 item scale combining items from the Rutter B scale and the Connors teacher rating scale.[12] No teacher behaviour ratings were available at 5 years.

Factor analysis of the maternally reported behaviour problem scale produced two first order subscales at age 5: antisocial and neurotic behaviour.[13] To allow for the possibility that otitis media affects specific aspects of behaviour, antisocial behaviour was broken down into two second order factors: (1) hyperactive behaviour with items including the child not concentrating, teasing other children, and being excitable, impulsive, restless, overactive, and easily distracted; and (2) behaviour associated with "poor conduct", characterised as destroying belongings, frequently fighting, taking things belonging to others, etc. This division might provide further insight into the specific types of behaviours associated with middle ear disease.

Similar subscales for maternal and teacher reported behaviour at age 10 were derived using factor analysis; these included antisocial and neurotic behaviour and clumsiness.[12] In addition, ratings of inattentiveness were recorded in the teacher scale and hyperactive behaviour in the maternal scale. Speech articulation was reported in an additional questionnaire covering the educational and social environment of the study child, as seen by the class teacher and school head.

Table 1 Prevalence (%) of behaviour problems at 5 years of age in relation to ear discharge, hearing difficulty, sex, and socioeconomic status

	Extreme antisocial behaviour (n)	Extreme neurotic behaviour (n)	Hyperactivity (n)	Poor conduct (n)
Ear discharge up to age 5				
Never	9.4 (1051)	9.5 (1055)	9.9 (1098)	9.6 (1066)
Ever	13.1 (190)	13.0 (188)	13.6 (196)	12.6 (182)
Hearing difficulty up to age 5				
Never	9.6 (1107)	9.6 (1107)	9.9 (1137)	9.7 (1115)
Ever	13.0 (137)	13.9 (147)	14.4 (151)	12.8 (135)
Sex				
Male	13.0 (883)	8.9 (605)	11.3 (765)	13.0 (883)
Female	6.7 (423)	11.1 (701)	9.4 (589)	6.7 (426)
Socioeconomic status of household				
1 (most advantaged)	4.0 (109)	9.2 (251)	6.5 (178)	5.3 (144)
2 (average)	8.9 (616)	9.4 (646)	9.7 (664)	8.9 (616)
3 (most disadvantaged)	16.6 (580)	11.6 (406)	14.8 (512)	15.8 (549)

All comparisons are significant, $p < 0.01$.

COGNITIVE TEST DATA

Verbal performance tests at 5 years included the English picture vocabulary test (EPVT), similar to the American Peabody picture vocabulary test, which is a test of passive vocabulary. Non-verbal tests at 5 years included human figure drawing (a modified version of the "draw a man" test measuring conceptual maturity) and the copy design test (CDT). In the CDT, children were asked to make two copies of each of eight designs, which were later judged blind on shape, symmetry, neatness, etc.

Verbal tests at 10 included a picture language score (similar to EPVT) and the verbal IQ British ability scales (BAS). Verbal BAS includes the three subtests: word definitions, recall of digits, and similarities, similar to those in the American differential ability scales (DAS). The non-verbal BAS measured at 10 years included the matrices test.

ANALYSES

On the continuous and normally distributed dependent measures (behaviour and cognitive tests) all effects were examined initially using analysis of covariance. In addition, for the behavioural scores only, binary variables were derived by defining a cut off at the 90th centile of the distribution to test the operative range of associations. A score falling beyond this extreme suggests a level of gross behaviour problems justifying concern. Overall, the two types of analysis gave similar patterns of results for the behaviour scores. Logistic regression analysis was used to examine the relation between the covariates and these binary behavioural variables. The ear discharge and hearing difficulty responses were considered separately as independent variables.

Adjusted odds ratios (OR) and 95% confidence intervals (CI) for behaviour problems in relation to middle ear disease were computed using logistic regression, controlling for sex, socioeconomic status, and maternal malaise at 5 years. An OR > 1 indicates that behaviour problems are more likely in the middle ear disease compared with the control group and an OR < 1 indicates that behavioural problems are less likely.

Results

The prevalences of middle ear disease in BCS70 are: 11.5% for ear discharge (probably reflecting the poorly treated extreme of acute otitis media in the 1970s) and 8.4% for hearing difficulty (probably reflecting cumulative OME severity and persistence of effusion), conforming to that found in objectively established epidemiological data.[14] In addition, we have shown highly significant mutual associations between the two markers and with the known otitis media risk factors (such as parental smoking and attendance at day care), consistent with the epidemiological literature.[15]

CONTRASTS AT 5 YEARS OF AGE

For the 5 year data, preliminary univariate analyses (raw relative risks) for the ear discharge and hearing difficulty variables with individual behaviour items have been reported elsewhere,[5] but prevalence figures for behaviour scores are given in table 1. To enhance reliability and generalisation, subscales from factor analysis are used here. We have reported elsewhere[16] preliminary main effect associations at age 5, for mean behaviour (antisocial and neurotic) scores only. For interpretation as sequelae, greater multivariate statistical control is presented here. All associations reported are in the direction of greater deficit or abnormality for the marker value reflecting a middle ear disease history.

Table 2 gives the mean magnitude (in SD units) of effects of ear discharge and hearing difficulty on the behaviours reported at 5 years. Overall, the effects of the adjustments made were mostly quite small. Taking the overall mean, the largest magnitude effects at 5 years are seen in the neurotic and hyperactive behaviours. Irrespective of middle ear disease, the prevalence of reported behavioural problems is higher in children with a more disadvantaged socioeconomic status (table 1), thus confirming the requirement for control of socioeconomic status.

Table 2 Unadjusted and adjusted magnitude of effects of hearing difficulty and ear discharge on the continuous behaviour scores at 5 years of age

Middle ear disease marker	Antisocial	Neurotic	Hyperactive	Poor conduct
Unadjusted magnitudes				
Hearing difficulty	0.13	0.22	0.19	0.08
Ear discharge	0.15	0.20	0.13	0.14
Adjusted* magnitudes and 95% CI				
Hearing difficulty	0.12 (0.06 to 0.18)	0.20 (0.14 to 0.25)	0.19 (0.12 to 0.25)	0.07 (0.01 to 0.13)
Ear discharge	0.08 (0.03 to 0.13)	0.14 (0.09 to 0.19)	0.07 (0.02 to 0.13)	0.07 (0.02 to 0.12)

Results are reported in SD units and are for parent reported behaviour (Rutter A scale).
*Adjusted for socioeconomic status, sex, and maternal malaise (n = 12 554).

Table 3 Unadjusted and adjusted odds ratio of dichotomous behaviour scores at 5 years of age as a function of ear discharge

Socioeconomic status (grouped)	*Antisocial*	*Neurotic*	*Hyperactivity*	*Poor conduct*
Unadjusted odds ratio				
1 (most advantaged)	2.01	1.46	1.24	1.55
2 (average)	1.27	1.41	1.41	1.21
3 (most disadvantaged)	1.49	1.40	1.48	1.41
Overall (95% CI)	1.45 (1.21 to 1.64)	1.43 (1.20 to 1.69)	1.42 (1.21 to 1.68)	1.35 (1.14 to 1.60)
Adjusted* odds ratio and 95% CI				
1 (most advantaged)	1.70 (1.03 to 2.78)	1.27 (0.86 to 1.87)	1.10 (0.70 to 1.74)	1.35 (0.85 to 2.15)
2 (average)	1.14 (0.87 to 1.48)	1.29 (1.01 to 1.66)	1.31 (1.03 to 1.68)	1.09 (0.84 to 1.43)
3 (most disadvantaged)	1.33 (1.02 to 1.74)	1.21 (0.89 to 1.65)	1.35 (1.03 to 1.77)	1.26 (0.96 to 1.65)
Overall†	1.27 (1.07 to 1.52)	1.27 (1.07 to 1.51)	1.29 (1.09 to 1.52)	1.19 (1.0 to 1.42)
p value for ear discharge	0.008	0.007	0.003	0.054

Results are for parent reported behaviour—defined at 90th centile of distribution of continuous scores.
*Adjusted for sex and maternal malaise. †Overall odds ratio (combining all socioeconomic status groups) adjusted for sex, socioeconomic status, and maternal malaise (n = 12 497).

Ear discharge
Antisocial, neurotic, and hyperactive behaviour dichotomised at the 90th centile were significantly associated with having had ear discharge, but behaviour associated with poor conduct was not. The overall ORs (table 3) were fairly uniform across the types of behaviour; antisocial behaviour shows some social trend, but this was not significant.

The verbal test (standardised EPVT), nonverbal test, copy design, and the human figure drawing test showed no significant effects of having had ear discharge.

Hearing difficulty
Antisocial, neurotic, hyperactive behaviour, and poor conduct behaviours were significantly associated with having had hearing difficulty (table 4). These effects were larger than those for ear discharge, with an increased odds of extreme problems (beyond the 90th centile) of about 50% in those having hearing difficulty (adjusted overall OR, 1.44 for antisocial and 1.52 for neurotic behaviour). A marginally significant interaction ($p = 0.06$) was found for hyperactive behaviour representing synergy of hearing difficulty with maternal malaise; those children having both hearing difficulty and mothers with high malaise scores scored higher. This provides some evidence of synergistic relations between middle ear disease and other aspects of the environment in producing outcomes, giving clues to possible mechanisms.[17] The verbal test (standardised EPVT) was significantly affected by reported hearing difficulty at 5 years ($p < 0.05$; effect size, 0.17 SD), after adjustments for socioeconomic status and maternal malaise, but no significant interactions were found. The nonverbal test, human figure drawing, showed a small but significant effect of having had hearing difficulty ($p = 0.01$; effect size, 0.12 SD), but no significant interactions. The copy design test showed no significant effect of having had hearing difficulty.

CONTRASTS AT 10 YEARS OF AGE
Tables 5 and 6 show the mean magnitude (in SD units) of effect and 95% CI of ear discharge and hearing difficulty on the parent and teacher reported behaviours at 10 years.

Other results from the 10 year behaviour data from both parent and teacher are summarised in tables 7–10 as ORs (with 95% CI) for

Table 4 Unadjusted and adjusted odds ratio of dichotomous behaviour scores at 5 years of age as a function of reported hearing difficult*

Socioeconomic status (grouped)	*Antisocial*	*Neurotic*	*Hyperactivity*	*Poor conduct*
Unadjusted odds ratio				
1 (most advantaged)	1.56	1.92	1.30	1.61
2 (average)	1.65	1.45	1.69	1.49
3 (most disadvantaged)	1.44	1.44	1.75	1.40
Overall (95% CI)	1.41 (1.20 to 1.70)	1.53 (1.27 to 1.80)	1.53 (1.27 to 1.84)	1.37 (1.13 to 1.66)
Adjusted* odds ratio and 95% CI				
1 (most advantaged)	1.55 (0.90 to 2.66)	2.05 (1.42 to 2.94)	1.29 (0.81 to 2.04)	1.61 (1.01 to 2.58)
2 (average)	1.26 (1.17 to 2.03)	1.36 (1.04 to 1.82)	1.61 (1.25 to 2.12)	1.40 (1.06 to 1.86)
3 (most disadvantaged)	1.25 (0.88 to 1.76)	1.36 (0.92 to 2.02)	1.62 (1.16 to 2.28)	1.23 (0.87 to 1.75)
Overall†	1.44 (1.18 to 1.76)	1.52 (1.26 to 1.85)	1.56 (1.29 to 1.89)	1.37 (1.12 to 1.67)
p value for hearing difficulty	0.001	0.000	0.000	0.003

Results are parent reported behaviour—defined at 90th centile of distribution of continuous scores.
*Adjusted for sex and maternal malaise. †Overall odds ratio (combining all socioeconomic status groups) adjusted for sex, socioeconomic status, and maternal malaise (n = 12 534).

Table 5 Effects of hearing difficulty and ear discharge on the continuous behaviour scores at 10 years of age—parent reported behaviour (Rutter A scale)

Middle ear disease marker	*Antisocial*	*Neurotic*	*Inattentive*	*Clumsy*
Unadjusted magnitudes				
Hearing difficulty	−0.05	0.15	0.23	0.07
Ear discharge	0.11	0.14	0.12	0.01
Adjusted* magnitudes and 95% CI				
Hearing difficulty	−0.01 (−0.07 to 0.06)	0.15 (0.08 to 0.22)	0.25 (0.18 to 0.32)	0.07 (0.004 to 0.14)
Ear discharge	0.10 (0.05 to 0.162)	0.14 (0.07 to 0.20)	0.11 (0.05 to 0.17)	0.01 (−0.04 to 0.07)

Results are in SD units.
*Adjusted for socioeconomic status only (n = 10 867).

Table 6 Effects of hearing difficulty and ear discharge on the continuous behaviour scores at 10 years of age—teacher reported behaviour (Rutter B scale)

Middle ear disease marker	Antisocial	Neurotic	Inattentive	Clumsy
Unadjusted magnitudes				
Hearing difficulty	0.11	0.12	−0.01	0.06
Ear discharge	0.10	0.09	0.09	0.070
Adjusted* magnitude and 95% CI				
Hearing difficulty	0.134 (0.06 to 0.21)	0.106 (0.03 to 0.18)	0.035 (−0.003 to 0.15)	0.071 (−0.04 to 011)
Ear discharge	0.108 (0.05 to 0.17)	0.081 (0.02 to 0.43)	0.072 (0.01 to 0.13)	0.069 (0.01 to 0.13)

Results are in SD units.
*Adjusted for socioeconomic status only (n = 9278).

the dichotomy at the 90th centile. Tables 7 and 9 indicate that behaviour problems at 10 years of age remain significantly associated with earlier reported ear/hearing problems.

Parental ratings: associations with ear discharge
The ORs for antisocial, neurotic, hyperactive, and clumsy behaviour all significantly reflected reported ear discharge (table 7), and were of a similar magnitude to those reported at 5 years. There was also a significant sex interaction (p = 0.01) in antisocial behaviour.

Parental ratings: associations with hearing difficulty
Reported hearing difficulty significantly raised the OR for neurotic, clumsy, and hyperactive behaviour but not for antisocial behaviour (table 9). Significant interactions were found in neurotic behaviour (p = 0.002, socioeconomic status by malaise; p = 0.03, sex by malaise), and in hyperactive behaviour (p = 0.002, sex by socioeconomic status). Although the interactions here do not involve the middle ear disease variable, they were considered important as they reflect the additional influence of synergies between the controlling variables.

The adjusted overall OR of 1.76 for hyperactive behaviour in the case of hearing difficulty is fairly large.

Teacher ratings
The teacher reported data (tables 8 and 10) show that antisocial behaviour is significantly associated with both ear discharge and hearing difficulty, but that neurotic and inattentive behaviour are not, and clumsy behaviour has only a marginal association. For antisocial behaviour, there was also a marginally significant interaction of hearing difficulty with socioeconomic status (p = 0.05). Clumsy behaviour was found to be significantly associated with hearing difficulty (p = 0.02; effect size, 0.08 SD), but not with ear discharge.

At 10 years, the verbal picture language test was significantly associated with ear discharge (p = 0.01; effect size, −0.08 SD); the negative sign indicates a deficit in language skills for children with reported ear discharge, but not with hearing difficulty. The verbal and non-verbal BAS were not significantly associated with either ear discharge or hearing difficulty. Speech articulation, as reported by the teacher, appeared significantly associated with a hearing

Table 7 Odds ratios for dichotomised parent reported behaviour scores at 10 years of age with ear discharge

Socioeconomic status (grouped)	Antisocial	Neurotic	Hyperactive	Clumsy
Unadjusted odds ratio				
1 (most advantaged)	1.24	1.27	1.57	1.44
2 (average)	1.28	1.34	1.45	1.50
3 (most disadvantaged)	1.41	1.42	1.35	0.95
Overall (95% CI)	1.36 (1.14 to 1.63)	1.35 (1.13 to 1.62)	1.45 (1.21 to 1.73)	1.31 (1.09 to 1.57)
Adjusted* odds ratio and 95% CI				
1 (most advantaged)	1.02 (0.75 to 1.82)	1.07 (0.70 to 1.64)	1.29 (0.83 to 2.02)	1.40 (0.94 to 2.09)
2 (average)	1.20 (0.90 to 1.59)	1.28 (0.99 to 1.66)	1.41 (1.10 to 1.81)	1.47 (1.14 to 1.89)
3 (most disadvantaged)	1.37 (1.04 to 1.81)	1.34 (0.95 to 1.88)	1.33 (0.97 to 1.83)	0.96 (0.61 to 1.37)
Overall†	1.26 (1.05 to 1.52)	1.26 (1.05 to 1.52)	1.37 (1.15 to 1.64)	1.29 (1.08 to 1.55)
p value for ear discharge	0.018	0.015	0.001	0.006

Results are Rutter A scale—defined at 90th centile of distribution of continuous scores.
*Adjusted for sex and maternal malaise. †Combining all socioeconomic status groups—adjusted for sex, socioeconomic status, and maternal malaise (n = 10 728).

Table 8 Odds ratios for dichotomised teacher reported behaviour scores at 10 years with ear discharge

Socioeconomic status (grouped)	Antisocial	Neurotic	Inattentive	Clumsy
Unadjusted odds ratio				
1 (most advantaged)	0.97	0.86	1.72	0.74
2 (average)	1.53	1.21	1.18	1.12
3 (most disadvantaged)	1.64	1.17	1.06	1.37
Overall (95% CI)	1.40 (1.16 to 1.68)	1.14 (0.93 to 1.38)	1.25 (1.03 to 1.52)	1.05 (0.86 to 1.28)
Adjusted* odds ratio and 95% CI				
1 (most advantaged)	0.88 (0.52 to 1.50)	0.80 (0.48 to 1.34)	1.55 (0.93 to 2.57)	0.77 (0.47 to 1.27)
2 (average)	1.51 (1.14 to 1.94)	1.15 (0.89 to 1.58)	1.13 (0.85 to 1.50)	1.14 (0.86 to 1.52)
3 (most disadvantaged)	1.76 (1.15 to 2.31)	1.16 (0.77 to 1.68)	1.06 (0.73 to 1.55)	1.34 (0.91 to 1.99)
Overall†	1.42 (1.17 to 1.73)	1.10 (0.89 to 1.35)	1.17 (0.95 to 1.44)	1.10 (0.90 to 1.36)
p value for ear discharge	0.001	0.402	0.166	0.356

Results are Rutter B scale—defined at 90th centile of distribution of continuous scores.
*Adjusted for sex and maternal malaise. †Combining all socioeconomic status groups—adjusted for sex, socioeconomic status, and maternal malaise (n = 9283).

Table 9 Odds ratios for dichotomised parent reported behaviour scores at 10 years with hearing difficulty

Socioeconomic status (grouped)	*Antisocial*	*Neurotic*	*Hyperactive*	*Clumsy*
Unadjusted odds ratio				
1 (most advantaged)	0.96	1.19	1.84	1.23
2 (average)	1.31	1.70	1.91	1.35
3 (most disadvantaged)	1.16	1.29	1.80	1.73
Overall (95% CI)	1.09 (0.87 to 1.36)	1.46 (1.19 to 1.79)	1.78 (1.47 to 2.16)	1.38 (1.12 to 1.69)
Adjusted* odds ratio and 95% CI				
1 (most advantaged)	0.88 (0.46 to 1.68)	1.12 (0.72 to 1.75)	1.69 (1.09 to 2.63)	1.21 (0.79 to 1.86)
2 (average)	1.15 (0.83 to 1.58)	1.55 (1.18 to 2.05)	1.77 (1.36 to 2.32)	1.28 (0.96 to 1.72)
3 (most disadvantaged)	1.05 (0.71 to 1.56)	1.29 (0.81 to 2.05)	1.72 (1.16 to 2.54)	1.68 (1.11 to 2.54)
Overall†	1.10 (0.87 to 1.38)	1.40 (1.14 to 1.72)	1.76 (1.45 to 2.14)	1.36 (1.10 to 1.67)
p value for hearing difficulty	0.522	0.002	0.000	0.004

Results are Rutter A scale—defined at 90th centile of distribution of continuous scores.
*Adjusted for sex and maternal malaise. †Combining all socioeconomic status groups—adjusted for sex, socioeconomic status, and maternal malaise (n = 10 750).

Table 10 Odds ratio for dichotomised teacher reported behaviour scores at 10 years with hearing difficulty

Socioeconomic status (grouped)	*Antisocial*	*Neurotic*	*Inattentive*	*Clumsy*
Unadjusted odds ratio				
1 (most advantaged)	0.73	1.38	1.06	1.61
2 (average)	1.66	0.99	1.34	0.87
3 (most disadvantaged)	1.62	1.89	0.72	2.01
Overall (95% CI)	1.30 (1.04 to 1.62)	1.20 (0.96 to 1.51)	1.06 (0.84 to 1.35)	1.23 (0.98 to 1.54)
Adjusted* odds ratio and 95% CI				
1 (most advantaged)	0.73 (0.40 to 1.35)	1.38 (0.87 to 2.19)	0.98 (0.53 to 1.81)	1.68 (1.12 to 2.53)
2 (average)	1.58 (1.18 to 2.12)	0.95 (0.68 to 1.35)	1.25 (0.92 to 1.70)	0.89 (0.62 to 1.27)
3 (most disadvantaged)	1.51 (0.96 to 2.38)	1.91 (1.22 to 2.99)	0.68 (0.39 to 1.21)	2.08 (1.32 to 3.28)
Overall†	1.38 (1.10 to 1.73)	1.25 (0.99 to 1.58)	1.07 (0.83 to 1.37)	1.31 (1.04 to 1.64)
p value for hearing difficulty	0.007	0.069	0.703	0.022

Results are for Rutter B scale—defined at 90th centile of distribution of continuous scores. Hearing difficulty by socioeconomic status interaction, p = 0.053.
*Adjusted for sex and maternal malaise. †Combining all socioeconomic status groups—adjusted for sex, socioeconomic status, and maternal malaise (n = 9324).

problem (p = 0.004; effect size, 0.13 SD) and with ear discharge (p = 0.048; effect size, 0.08 SD). All of these effects are relatively small.

The effects of reported ear discharge on the non-verbal and verbal BAS, although non-significant, were in the expected direction of slightly higher scores without discharge compared with those with discharge. On the non-verbal and verbal tests, the scores for those with reported hearing difficulty did not differ from those without.

Discussion

Recent research reviews[2 18] of otitis media developmental sequelae have highlighted the methodological difficulties and have recommended appropriate research designs. However, the gradually accumulating pattern of results in the larger and better controlled studies makes it increasingly difficult to doubt that there are OME sequelae in cognition and behaviour, although some authors[19] continue to question that such sequelae exist.

This analysis of a large national cohort extends the age range of associations reported because it has enough power to detect modest differences and provide the relevant statistical control (although in many cases this only makes a modest difference). Our analyses have shown a consistent set of effects in the behavioural scores of children by teachers as well as parents across both the ear discharge and hearing difficulty markers, suggesting that the effects from ear disease histories, as reflected by such markers, are genuine although small. Broadly, we find fewer associations with middle ear disease at 10 years than 5 years, as expected from remission of histories and the accumulation of other sources of variance.

A number of studies have considered the accuracy of parental reporting of children's disease histories.[9 20] They show that parental reporting can be fairly accurate compared with medical records, but it can be influenced by chronicity, duration of recall, and seriousness of the event.

INTERPRETATION OF PATTERNS OF RESULTS

Control for confounders

Special purpose studies can afford to include measurements that can be used to control for bias in parents' noticing both their child's health status and behavioural problems. The main reason for not believing such a possible source of artefact to be important here lies in the generally similar magnitude and pattern of results obtained when substituting ear discharge for hearing difficulty as the independent variable; we know from the analysis of socioeconomic status that hearing difficulty is subject to cultural reporting biases, but ear discharge is not. Yet, even if socioeconomic status is adjusted for, the sequelae effects found for ear discharge are no weaker overall than those for hearing difficulty, suggesting no socioeconomic status artefact. It is recognised in our analysis that statistical adjustment for socioeconomic status may not fully capture the cultural variables influencing measured abilities thereby resulting in incomplete adjustment.

The second reason for rejecting interpretation in terms of response bias is that we find comparable results from the teacher reported data, which have greater objectivity and power.

Although the degree of control exercised here is sufficient to rule out major confounders, it does not permit all of the effects to be ascribed to particular paths of developmental influences as in the arrows of fig 1.

Behavioural sequelae
Persistent OME in early childhood, leading to prolonged auditory deprivation, appears to lead to various behaviour problems at 5 and 10 years of age. These comprise inattentive or hyperactive, antisocial, and neurotic behaviours. Behaviour problems associated with middle ear disease could come about in several ways. The main possibility is difficulty with human communication, as a result of not being able to hear properly, as mentioned earlier.[1] Other processes, mediated by generally lowered motivation and non-specific illness could also influence the behaviours reported here—for example, the child becoming withdrawn or neurotic.

Among cohort studies, only the Dunedin study[6 21] has published data on otitis media and behaviour problems. At age 5 years, 69 of the 1037 cohort members had bilateral type B tympanograms or ventilation tubes in situ. They had significantly more teacher reported behaviour problems than those with normal hearing. At ages 11 and 13, lower verbal IQ and parent and teacher reports of inattentive behaviour were associated significantly with an early history of OME.[21] However, the sample was not large enough, and the main socioeconomic gradient was too slight to test and control for interactions of OME status with socioeconomic group.

The epidemiological finding of clumsy behaviour associated with middle ear disease adds to clinical research,[22 23] suggesting possible vestibular side effects of middle ear disease. The Dunedin study[21] found deficits of motor skills from a history of middle ear disease. These unexpected deficits could be caused by vestibular dysfunction or by other factors, such as the "illness effect" of a history of upper respiratory tract infection, or to some systemic neuroimmunological factor.

Language and cognitive deficits
In the Dunedin cohort, children with bilateral OME were found to have significantly lower scores in intelligence, motor skills, verbal comprehension, and verbal expression than normal hearing children, but not in speech articulation, at 5 years. The Nijmegen longitudinal population study of 1328 children[7] found some association between OME and language development in preschool children, but this had disappeared by school age (7–8 years). This suggests short lived effects for language deficits, in line with most of the findings of more intensively studied small samples. The Boston study[8] tested speech and language in 205 children aged 3 years from a practice based cohort of 698, comparing those with little or no history of OME to those with a prolonged history. Scores were lower on receptive/expressive language, speech articulation, complexity of language, and intelligibility. By 7 years, there were still some significant associations for intelligence, speech/language, and school performance.[24]

Most of these published studies of otitis media developmental sequelae involve children young enough to show some effect of middle ear history on language delay.[25] This does not mean that all language effects in older children must be null. In a large sample with adequate control for socioeconomic status and maternal malaise, our analysis suggests that, at 10 years of age, there is a small reduction in active vocabulary associated with middle ear disease. We interpret this small effect size as consistent with transient language effects undergoing "catch up" from partial hearing or on eventual remission. An early language effect might influence the substrate of later educational achievement plus the cognitive and emotional development of the child. Further studies are required to distinguish these possibilities, but overall the conclusion remains that by school age formal language difficulties are more subtle and harder to show.

INTERVENTIONS
Our data provide a benchmark (a modest 0.2 SD) for the mean magnitude of otitis media sequelae, and indicate that clinical trials seeking to show reductions in sequelae by surgical intervention would need to be very large.

An alternative view of effects around 0.2 SD is that about 5% of all children (that is, half the materially affected children) have effects larger than this, so our conclusions for the general case do not mean that otitis media is universally benign. Parental and teacher awareness and close monitoring is required in all cases, as is intervention in extreme cases (surgical treatment or behavioural management). Criteria for referral to speech and language therapists or psychologists would need to be formulated and tested in trials. As with medical interventions, the problem of structuring and specifying the interventions of the various professionals involved, to ensure that they are efficacious and amenable to rigorous evaluation for effectiveness, will be great.

We are grateful to the social statistics research unit at City University, London for supplying the documented data and to the Hearing Research Trust for supplementary financial support (Defeating Deafness).

1 Roberts JE and Schuele C. Otitis media and later academic performance: the linkage and implications for intervention. *Topics in Language Disorder* 1990;11:43–62.
2 Teele D.W. Long term sequelae of otitis media: fact or fantasy? *Pediatr Infect Dis J* 1994;13:1069–73.
3 Wallace IF, Gravel JS, Schwartz RG, Ruben RJ. Otitis media, communication style of primary caregivers, and language skills of 2 year olds: a preliminary report. *J Dev Behav Pediatr* 1996;17:27–35.
4 Rutter M. Commentary: some focus and process considerations regarding effects of parental depression on children. *Dev Psychol* 1990;26:60–7.
5 Butler NR, Golding J. *From birth to five.* Oxford: Pergamon Press, 1986.
6 Silva P, Kirkland C, Simpson A, Stewart A, Williams SM. Some developmental and behavioural problems associated with bilateral otitis media with effusion. *J Learn Disabil* 1984;15:417–21.
7 Schilder AGM, van Manen JG, Zielhuis G, Grievink E, Peters S, van den Broek P. Long-term effects of otitis media with effusion on language, reading and spelling. *Clin Otolaryngol* 1993;18:234–41.
8 Teele DW, Klein JO, Rosner BA, and the Greater Boston Otitis Media Study Group. Otitis media with effusion during the first three years of life and development of speech and language. *Pediatrics* 1984;74:282–7.

9 Daly KA, Lindgren B, Giebink G.S. Validity of parental eport of a child's medical history in otitis media research. *Am J Epidemiol* 1994;**139**:1116–21.
10 Osborn AF. Assessing the socio-economic status of families. *Sociology* 1987;**21**:429–48.
11 Rutter M, Tizard J, Whitmore K. *Education, health and behaviour*. London: Longman, 1970.
12 Butler NR, Haslum MN, Barker W, Morris AC. *Child health and education study. First report to the Department of Education and Science on the 10-year follow-up*. Department of Child Health, University of Bristol, 1982.
13 Osborn AF, Butler NR, Morris AC. *The social life of Britain's five-year-olds*. London: Routledge and Kegan Paul, 1984.
14 Zielhuis GA, Rach GH, Van den Bosch A, Van den Broek P. The prevalance of otitis media wih effusion. A critical review of the literature. *Clin Otolaryngol* 1990;**15**:283–8.
15 Bennett KE, Haggard MP. Accumulation of factors influencing children's middle ear disease—risk factor modelling on a large population cohort. *J Epidemiol Community Health*. [In press.]
16 Haggard MP, Birkin JA, Browning GG, Gatehouse S, Lewis S. Behaviour problems in otitis media. *Pediatr Infect Dis J* 1994;**13**:S43–50.
17 Gortmaker SL, Walker DK, Weitzman M, Sobol AM. Chronic conditions, socioeconomic risks, and behavioural problems in children and adolescents. *Pediatrics* 1990;**85**: 267–76.
18 Paradise JL. Does early-life otitis media result in lasting developmental impairment? Why the question persists, and a proposed plan for addressing it. *Adv Pediatr* 1992;**39**:157–65.
19 Roberts JE, Burchinal MR, Davis BP, Collier AM, Henderson FW. Otitis media in early childhood and later language. *J Speech Hear Res* 1992;**34**:1158–68.
20 Pless CE, Pless IB. How well they remember—the accuracy of parent reports. *Arch Pediatr Adolesc Med* 1995;**149**:553–8.
21 Chalmers D, Stewart IA, Silva PA, Mulvena M. *Otitis media with effusion in children—the Dunedin study*. Oxford: Blackwell, 1989.
22 Jones NS, Prichard AJN, Radomshij P, Snashall SE. Imbalance and chronic secretory otitis media in children: effect of myringotomy and insertion of ventilation tubes on body sway. *Ann Otol Rhinol Laryngol* 1990;**99**:477–81.
23 Casselbrant ML, Gurman JM, Rubenstein E, Mandel EM. Effects of otitis media on the vestibular system in children. *Ann Otol Rhinol Laryngol* 1995;**104**:620–4.
24 Teele DW, Klein JO, Chase C, Menyuk P, Rosner BA, and the Greater Boston Otitis Media Study Group. Otitis media in infancy and intellectual ability, school achievement, speech and language at age 7 years. *J Infect Dis* 1990; **162**:685–94.
25 Friel-Patti S, Finitzo T, Formby E, Brown KC. A prospective study of early middle ear disease and speech-language development. *Texas Journal of Audiology and Speech Pathology* 1987;**13**:39–42.

PROGNOSIS WORKSHEET: 1 of 2

Clinical question:

Are the results of this prognosis study valid?

Was a defined, representative sample of patients assembled at a common (usually early) point in the course of their disease?

Was patient follow-up sufficiently long and complete?

Were objective outcome criteria applied in a 'blind' fashion?

If subgroups with different prognoses are identified, was there adjustment for important prognostic factors?

Was there validation in an independent group ('test-set') of patients?

Are the valid results of this prognosis study important?

How likely are the outcomes over time?

How precise are the prognostic estimates?

If you want to calculate a Confidence Interval around the measure of Prognosis

see Appendix 1 in *Evidence-based Medicine*.

Clinical measure	Standard error (SE)	Typical calculation of CI
Proportion (as in the rate of some prognostic event, etc.) where: the number of patients = n the proportion of these patients who experience the event = p	$\sqrt{\{p \times (1 - p) / n\}}$ where p is proportion and n is number of patients	If p = 24/60 = 0.4 (or 40%) & n = 60 SE = $\sqrt{\{0.4 \times (1 - 0.4) / 60\}}$ = 0.063 (or 6.3%) 95% CI is 40% +/– 1.96 × 6.3% or 27.6% to 52.4%
n from your evidence: ________ p from your evidence: ________	$\sqrt{\{p \times (1 - p) / n\}}$ where p is proportion and n is number of patients	Your calculation: SE: ____________ 95% CI:

Can you apply this valid, important evidence about prognosis in caring for your patient?

Were the study patients similar to your own?

Will this evidence make a clinically important impact on your conclusions about what to offer or tell your patient?

Additional notes

COMPLETED PROGNOSIS WORKSHEET: 1 of 2

Clinical question: Are children with middle ear disease at increased risk of behavioural problems?

Are the results of this prognosis study valid?	
Was a defined, representative sample of patients assembled at a common (usually early) point in the course of their disease?	**Yes. Large birth cohort of more than 12 000.**
Was patient follow-up sufficiently long and complete?	**Maybe. Follow up was for 10 years. Original number stated as more than 12 000, at 5 years about 12 000 and at 10 years about 9000. Authors comment that the prevalance of middle ear disease was similar in children followed as in those lost to follow up but no figures given.**
Were objective outcome criteria applied in a 'blind' fashion?	**Yes. Scales for behaviour and cognitive ability based on parent and teacher responses to questions. Respondents were not necessarily blind to middle ear disease but many factors were studied, and therefore, unlikely to be affected.**
If subgroups with different prognoses are identified, was there adjustment for important prognostic factors?	**Yes. Adjustment for social class and maternal malaise, but may be incomplete. No other social or cultural factors, such as maternal age or education, taken into account.**
Was there validation in an independent group ('test-set') of patients?	**No, but previous cohort studies have reported a possible association.**

COMPLETED PROGNOSIS WORKSHEET: 2 of 2

Are the valid results of this prognosis study important?	
How likely are the outcomes over time?	**Look at risk of neurotic behaviour score greater than 90th centile at 10 years for children with hearing difficulty based on parent reports (Table 9). OR = 1.40 and for teacher reported behaviour (Table 10) OR = 1.25.** **However, using continuous variables, for parent reported behaviour the largest difference was for hyperactive behaviour, with a 0.25 SD difference at 10 years. This is small, and unlikely to be clinically important.**
How precise are the prognostic estimates?	**Can look at 95% confidence intervals around the odds ratio. CI around OR does not include 1 so result is statistically significant.** **OR for HD = 1.38 (1.1 to 1.73)** **OR for ED = 1.42 (1.17 to 1.73)**

Can you apply this valid, important evidence about prognosis in caring for your patient?	
Were the study patients similar to your own?	**Yes.**
Will this evidence make a clinically important impact on your conclusions about what to offer or tell your patient?	**Yes. Magnitude of effect is small but there is an association. Not enough information to discuss surgery as no evidence that intervention will alter long-term risks.**

Additional notes

1 The health visitor would probably advise the mother to inform the school when Liam has ear discharge or hearing difficulty, so teachers make an extra effort.
2 Surgery has not proven to reduce the behavioural or cognitive problems associated with glue ear, so cost of private surgery probably not warranted without more evidence.
3 The small difference in behaviour may nevertheless be important at a population level.
4 There is some suggestion of an interaction between social class and the effects of glue ear on behavioural and cognitive problems.

UNCERTAINTY PERSISTS WHETHER MIDDLE EAR DISEASE IN EARLY CHILDHOOD INCREASES THE RISK OF BEHAVIOUR PROBLEMS AT 10 YEARS

Appraised by R Gilbert:
4 March 1999
Expiry date: March 2000.

Clinical Bottom Line

Middle ear disease is associated with a small increase in behaviour problems at 10 years but the difference may not be clinically significant and may be partly explained by socio-economic factors.

Citation

Bennett KE and Haggard MP (1999) Behaviour and cognitive outcomes from middle ear disease. *Arch Dis Child* **80:** 28–35.

Clinical Question

Are children with middle ear disease at increased risk of behaviour problems?

The Study

1 Large, national birth cohort of 12 000 children.
2 Middle ear disease (discharge or hearing difficulty) and behaviour measured at 5 and 10 years by parental responses to questions and child assessment. Behaviour at 10 years also measured by teacher responses.
3 Follow up of about 12 000 at 5 years and about 9000 at 10 years. Authors state that loss to follow up did not significantly affect proportions that had middle ear disease.

The Evidence

Difference in behaviour score (measured in SD units) for children with reported hearing difficultly (adjusted for socio-economic status, 95% confidence interval)

	Antisocial	Neurotic	Hyperactive	Poor conduct
@ 5 years (parent reported)	0.12 (0.06 to 0.18)	0.20 (0.14–0.25)	0.19 (0.12–0.25)	0.07 (0.01–0.13)
@ 10 years (parent reported)	–0.01 (–0.07 to 0.06)	0.15 (0.08–0.22)	0.25 (0.18–0.32)	0.07 (0.00–0.14)

Comments

1 The differences in behaviour score are small. However, middle ear disease is common (10% in this cohort) and at a population level, these small differences may be clinically important.
2 The slightly higher adverse behaviour scores in children with hearing difficulty could be partly explained by residual confounding due to socio-economic factors.
3 Occurr ence of middle ear disease was based on parental reports and misclassification of exposure was likely. This may reduce the strength of true associations.

SOURCES OF EVIDENCE FOR EVIDENCE-BASED MEDICINE

Title	Medium	Content type	Advantages	Disadvantages
***Best Evidence* on disk (American College of Physicians & BMJ Publications Group)**	CD-ROM or diskette (cumulated contents of two paper journals: *ACP Journal Club* and *Evidence-based Medicine*). Updated every year.	Structured abstracts of articles from selected journals in internal medicine, general practice, obstetrics and gynaecology, paediatrics, psychiatry, and surgery. Articles must meet strict quality criteria; each abstract (evidence) accompanied by a commentary (clinical expertise).	High quality evidence with commentary; easy to search; high specificity (not much time wasted with irrelevant material).	Incomplete coverage of literature: low sensitivity.
WHEN TO USE IT: *As your first port of call for the specialities it covers.*				
Cochrane Library	CD-ROM or diskette or Internet	Superb evidence about therapy & prevention; thousands of world-wide systematic reviews; abstracts of overviews of effectiveness.	Highest-quality evidence we'll ever have on the effectiveness of health care.	Not yet many Cochrane reviews; necessarily omits the newest treatments.
WHEN TO USE IT: *As your best port of call for therapy.*				
MEDLINE (US National Library of Medicine)	Networked CD-ROM systems; on-line vendors. (SilverPlatter [WinSPIRS] Ovid, etc.)	Bibliographic records, with abstract and MeSH terms. Full-text services starting to appear.	Exhaustiveness; flexibility of searching; journal coverage; currency (on-line versions); widespread availability and support (lots of people can help you!)	Have to do your own quality filtering; putting together good searches is difficult; gaps in coverage (medical, geographical and linguistic).
WHEN TO USE IT: *When you need to be sure you've got everything and have time to search properly.*				
World-Wide Web (WWW, the Web, W3)	Internet (via browser programs such as Netscape, MS Internet Explorer, Mosaic, Yahoo, Lynx, etc.)	Everything: from LRs to NNTs; electronic journals (e.g. Bandolier) & journal clubs; software tools; CATs; teaching materials; searching tips; events and conferences; etc.	Some sites are excellent, with high-quality pre-filtered evidence; some good, free software; boundless possibilities; can be updated instantly.	Variable levels of quality control; poor sensitivity and specificity; access from NHS networks can be problematic; can be slow to download.
WHEN TO USE IT: *Find good sites and check them regularly for updates.*				
Recommended sites:	NHS R&D Centre for Evidence-based Medicine	http://cebm.jr2.ox.ac.uk/	CATs, NNTs, LRs, etc., teaching materials, announcements, links to other sites.	
	SCHARR / AurACLE	http://www.shef.ac.uk/~scharr/ir/netting.html	Evidence-based information seeking, links to other sites.	
	Bandolier	http://www.jr2.ox.ac.uk/Bandolier/	An electronic version (including back issues) of the EBM journal *Bandolier*.	
WWW search services	General comment on Web searching	Allow you to type in keywords and search an index of WWW pages.	Tens of millions of pages are indexed and can be accessed directly. Searching is crude and hits displayed in an order which is not always appropriate.	
Typical specific services:	Yahoo!	http://www.yahoo.com	More selective than most search sites, though this may not coincide with your needs!	
	AltaVista	http://www.altavista.com	Seems to be the most exhaustive, with best searching engine.	
WHEN TO USE IT: *To find very specific information from the Web or starting points for browsing.*				

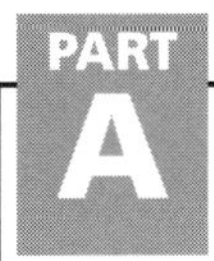

Critical appraisal of a systematic review

EBCH SESSION

4

SECTION 1

Systematic reviews and searching the primary literature

Section 1: Home visiting and child accident prevention

You are the practice manager in an inner city practice. The practice health visitor is about to retire, and you are considering whether to reallocate the resources to other services within the practice. The health visitor claims that she plays an important role in accident prevention and shows you the attached systematic review as evidence. You are aware that 5% of your childhood population (<5 years) suffer from accidental injuries.

What recommendations do you make to the practice management committee report about whether to continue to employ a health visitor in the practice? You formulate the question, in children can home visiting reduce the injury rate?

Search strategy for health visitors

Type in:
1 explode CHILD/ all subheadings
2 VISIT*
3 SYSTEMATIC*
4 REVIEW*
5 OVERVIEW*
6 REVIEW* OR OVERVIEW*
7 and #2 and (#3 and #6)

You find the enclosed article (*BMJ* 1996; **312:** 29–33).

Read the systematic review and decide:
1 Is the evidence from this systematic review valid?
2 Is this valid evidence from this systematic review important?
3 Can you apply this valid and important evidence from this systematic review in caring for your patient?

If you want to read some strategies for answering these sorts of questions, you could have a look at pp 97–9, 140–1 and 166–72 in *Evidence-based Medicine*.

PART B

Searching the primary literature

Colleagues from the library will come and whet your appetite for learning how to search for evidence in the clinical literature or hone the searching skills you already have developed. So bring along the clinical questions you generated in Session 2 (or any that you have generated in the meantime). Efficient EBM searching strategies that trade-off the sensitivity and specificity of your searches are on the next page.

If you haven't already done your search for your presentation in Sessions 6 and 7, now would be a good time to do it!

BEST SINGLE TERMS AND COMBINATIONS FOR HIGH SENSITIVITY MEDLINE SEARCHES ON THE BEST STUDIES OF TREATMENT, DIAGNOSIS, PROGNOSIS, OR CAUSE.

Search strategy	Sensitivity[1]	Specificity	Precision
For studies of treatment:			
Clinical trial (pt)	0.93	0.92	0.49
Randomised controlled trial (pt) or Drug therapy (sh) or Therapeutic use (sh) or Random: (tw)	0.99	0.74	0.22
For studies of prognosis:			
Exp cohort studies	0.60	0.80	0.11
Incidence or Exp mortality or Follow up studies or Mortality: (sh) or Prognosis: (tw) or Predict: (tw) or Course (tw)	0.92	0.73	0.11
For studies of aetiology or cause:			
Risk (tw)	0.67	0.79	0.15
Exp cohort studies or Exp risk or Odds and ratio: (tw) or Relative and risk: (tw) or Case and control: (tw)	0.82	0.70	0.14
For studies of diagnosis:			
Diagnosis (pe)	0.80	0.77	0.09
Exp Sensitivity and specificity or Diagnosis: (pe) or Diagnostic use or Sensitivity: (tw) or Specificity: (tw)	0.92	0.73	0.09

[1]**Sensitivity**, as defined in the study on which the table is based, is the proportion of studies in MEDLINE meeting criteria for scientific soundness and clinical relevance that are detected. **Specificity** is the proportion of less sound/relevant studies that are excluded by the search strategy. **Precision** is the proportion of all citations retrieved that are both sound and relevant (source: *Evidence-based Medicine*; see also the Web pages).

GENERAL PRACTICE

Does home visiting prevent childhood injury? A systematic review of randomised controlled trials

Ian Roberts, Michael S Kramer, Samy Suissa

Abstract

Objective—To quantify the effectiveness of home visiting programmes in the prevention of child injury and child abuse.

Design—Systematic review of 11 randomised controlled trials of home visiting programmes. Pooled odds ratios were estimated as an inverse variance weighted average of the study specific odds ratios.

Setting—Randomised trials that were available by April 1995.

Subjects—The trials comprised 3433 participants.

Results—Eight trials examined the effectiveness of home visiting in the prevention of childhood injury. The pooled odds ratio for the eight trials was 0·74 (95% confidence interval 0·60 to 0·92). Four studies examined the effect of home visiting on injury in the first year of life. The pooled odds ratio was 0·98 (0·62 to 1·53). Nine trials examined the effect of home visiting on the occurrence of suspected abuse, reported abuse, or out of home placement for child abuse. Because of the potential for bias in outcome reporting in these studies, pooled effect estimates were not calculated.

Conclusions—Home visiting programmes have the potential to reduce significantly the rates of childhood injury. The problem of differential surveillance for child abuse between intervention and control groups precludes the use of reported abuse as a valid outcome measure in controlled trials of home visiting.

Department of Community Paediatric Research, Montreal Children's Hospital, McGill University Faculty of Medicine, Montreal, Quebec, Canada
Ian Roberts, *overseas fellow*

Departments of Pediatrics and of Epidemiology and Biostatistics, McGill University Faculty of Medicine
Michael S Kramer, *professor*

Division of Clinical Epidemiology, Royal Victoria Hospital, Montreal
Samy Suissa, *director*

Correspondence to: Dr Ian Roberts, Department of Epidemiology and Biostatistics, Institute of Child Health, London WC1N 1EH.

BMJ 1996;312:29-33

Introduction

Home visiting programmes have long been advocated for improving the health of disadvantaged children. In Britain home visits by health visitors are considered to have a key role in accident prevention because of the advice given during the visits on child development and home safety.[1] In the United States home visiting has been promoted primarily for the prevention of child abuse and neglect.[2] In 1991 the United States Advisory Board on Child Abuse and Neglect called for the establishment of a universal programme of home visiting in an attempt to stem the increase in numbers of child abuse reports.[3]

Over the past two decades several randomised trials have examined the effect of home visiting programmes on the occurrence of child abuse and other child health outcomes. The results of these trials, however, have been conflicting. Although several published articles have reviewed the evidence from randomised trials,[4,5] none of these satisfies the methodological criteria that have been proposed for scientific overviews.[6] To quantify the effect of home visiting programmes on the occurrence of child injury and abuse we conducted a systematic review.

Methods

Inclusion criteria—We included studies in the systematic review if they met all three of the following criteria: (*a*) the assignment of the study participants to the intervention or control group had to be random or quasi-random—for example, alternate record numbers; (*b*) the study intervention had to include one or more postnatal home visits; and (*c*) the study had to address the outcomes of child injury (unintentional or intentional).

Identification of relevant trials—We identified trials by a computerised literature search of Medline (January 1966 to April 1995) and Embase (January 1975 to April 1995). We also searched the social sciences citation index for articles referencing randomised trials of home visiting. Key terms used for searching included social support, family support, home (and health) visitors, home (and health) visitation, child abuse, and child neglect. We reviewed the references of all relevant papers found in the searches, as well as those of review articles and textbooks. Because home visiting is often encountered in the context of the prevention of child abuse, a hand search was conducted of the *Journal of Child Abuse and Neglect* (from 1977 1(1) through to 1995 19(3)). We contacted the authors of identified papers and experts in the field and asked about any published or unpublished work that they might be aware of. To access studies not formally published, such as research reports and abstracts, we searched relevant conference proceedings. If studies met the first two inclusion criteria but did not report outcomes of child injury or abuse we asked the authors to provide any unpublished data on child injury.

Data extraction and study appraisal—We extracted the following data from each study: strategy for allocation concealment, number of randomised participants, duration of follow up, loss to follow up, blinding of outcome assessment, and the professional background of the home visitor (health or welfare professional or non-professional). We evaluated the quality of the trial using a modification of Prendiville's criteria.[7] With this approach trials are scored from 1 to 3 (1 - poorest score, 3 - best score) on three important aspects of study methodology: control of confounding at entry (adequacy of allocation concealment); control of selection bias (extent to which analyses are based on all randomised participants); and control of information bias in assessing outcome (blinding of observers). While the original criteria assigned a score of 3 for random assignment by telephone and 2 for using opaque sealed envelopes, we assigned a score of 3 for using either of these methods. Trials that assigned subjects to treatment by using methods intended to reduce the risk of foreknowledge of allocation but which were not as secure as random assignment by telephone or use of opaque sealed envelopes scored 2. Trials in which the authors did not report the method of allocation concealment (and were unable to provide further details or could not be contacted) and trials using alternate record numbers or other similar strategies scored 1. If a published report contained insufficient information for us to assess the quality of the trial, we asked the authors to provide further details. Two assessors performed the data extraction independently, with agreement on methodological criteria evaluated with weighted κ.[8] Each point of disagreement was settled by collaborative review.

Statistical methods—The measure of association, the odds ratio, was calculated directly for studies in which injury was expressed in binary (yes/no) form, with the variance estimated by Wolf's method.[9] For studies in which injury occurrence was allowed to be multiple and expressed as an incidence density, the odds ratio was estimated on the assumption of a Poisson distribution, with the probability of a participant having at least one event being given by $1-e^{-ID}$, where ID is the incidence density. Pooled odds ratios were then calculated as an inverse variance weighted average of the study specific odds ratios.

Results

The combined search strategies identified 33 trials meeting the first two inclusion criteria (randomised trials of postnatal home visiting).[10-42] Eleven of these trials (with 3433 participants) reported outcome data on injury or abuse, or on both.[10-19, 43] One of the eleven trials was published as an abstract only[42]; the author of this report was contacted, but the relevant outcome data were not available for inclusion in the review. Of the remaining 10 trials, one reported no differences in the occurrence of accidents,[13] and in another injury outcome data had been collected but not reported.[19] In both of these trials the authors gave us the relevant data. The authors of 13 of the 22 trials meeting the first two inclusion criteria but not reporting outcome data on injury or abuse responded to our request for information on unpublished injury outcomes. As a result of this process one further trial was identified that met all three inclusion criteria.[43] Eleven trials were therefore identified that had outcome data on injury or abuse, or both.

Table 1 shows the scores for the quality of methodology for the trials included in the systematic review. The weighted κ for agreement between the two assessors was 0·94 for adequacy of allocation concealment, 0·51 for the extent to which analyses were based on all randomised participants, and 0·78 for blinding. The mean scores for the unintentional injury outcomes were: adequacy of allocation concealment, 2·4; extent to which analyses were based on all randomised participants, 1·9; blinding, 1·5.

Child injury

Table 2 shows the data for the eight trials that examined the effect of home visiting on the occurrence of childhood injury. Six of the eight trials reported a lower incidence of injury in the group that received home visits. One study reported three injury outcome measures, representing three different time periods of follow up. For this study, the overall injury rates and odds ratios were calculated for the entire (four year) follow up period (odds ratio 0·74 (95% confidence interval 0·55 to 0·99)). The pooled odds ratio for injury for the eight trials (figure) was 0·74 (0·60 to 0·92). Four studies examined the effect of home visiting on injury occurrence in the first year of life only. The pooled odds ratio was 0·98 (0·62 to 1·53).

Child abuse

Table 3 shows the data for the nine trials that examined the effect of home visiting on the occurrence of suspected abuse, reported abuse, or out of home placement for child abuse. In four trials the frequency of occurrence of abuse was lower in the visited group. In five trials the frequency of occurrence was higher in the visited group. Substantial heterogeneity of the odds ratios was found across the studies. The potential for bias in the outcome reporting was considered to be a serious threat to validity in all nine studies. Specifically, the presence of the home visitor may have resulted in an increased surveillance for child abuse and hence an increase in the number of reports of abuse. If present, this bias would have resulted in an apparent increased incidence of abuse in the visited group. Pooled effect estimates were therefore not calculated.

Discussion

Although home visiting is unlikely to be associated with adverse effects, the widespread implementation or intensification of home visiting programmes may have important resource implications. Our meta-analysis of the results from eight randomised trials shows a significant preventive effect of home visiting on the occurrence of childhood injury.

Methodological issues

The effect of home visiting on the occurrence of child abuse varied across studies in both magnitude and direction. This may have been the result of bias in the assessment of child abuse outcomes. A report of child abuse entails the occurrence and discovery of an injury, as well as an attribution of intent. In several of the primary studies the information leading to the report of child abuse was provided by the home visitor, raising the possibility of "surveillance bias." Differential surveillance for child abuse between the inter-

Table 1—*Scores* for quality of methodology and study characteristics for randomised trials of home visiting*

Trial (year, country)	Allocation concealment	Analysed as randomised†	Blinding†	No of participants randomised	Follow up (years)
IHDP (1995, USA)	3	2	1	985	1
Marcenko *et al* (1994, USA)	2	2	1	225	0·8
Johnson *et al* (1994, Republic of Ireland)	3	2	1	262	1
Barth (1991, USA)	1	2	1	313	3
Dawson *et al* (1989, USA)	1	1	1	145	1
Hardy *et al* (1989, USA)	1	2	2	290	1·9
Olds *et al* (1986, USA)	3	1	2	400	4
Lealman *et al* (1983, England)	3	2	3	312	1·5
Larson (1980, Canada)	3	2	2	80	1·5
Siegel *et al* (1980, USA)	3	3	1	321	1
Gray *et al* (1979, USA)	3	2	1	100	1·4

IHDP–infant health and development programme.
*On scale of 1 to 3 (1–poorest score, 3–best score).
†Judged for injury outcome measures whenever possible.

Table 2—*Home visiting and childhood injury*

Trial (year, country)	Study population	Intervention	Outcome	Participants visited	Controls	Odds ratio (95% confidence interval)
IHDP (1995, USA)	Parents of low birthweight premature infants	Postnatal, non-professional, emotional, social, practical, and informational support	"Non-hospitalised injuries by maternal report"	17/345	26/551	1·05 (0·56 to 1·96)
Johnson *et al* (1993, Republic of Ireland)	Disadvantaged first time mothers	Postnatal, non-professional support and encouragement in child rearing using the child development programme	"Suffered an accident"	3/127	8/105	0·29 (0·08 to 1·14)
Hardy *et al* (1989, USA)	Inner city mothers of poor infants	Postnatal, non-professional parenting and childcare education	"Outpatient diagnosis of closed head trauma	8/131	15/132	0·51 (0·21 to 1·24)
Dawson *et al* (1989, USA)	Pregnant women attending for maternity care not selected for psychosocial risk	Antenatal and postnatal, non-professional emotional support; information and help in using community resources	"Accidents or ingestion requiring medical attention	5/67	6/44	0·51 (0·15 to 1·79)
Olds *et al* (1986, USA)	Primiparas who were teenagers, unmarried, or of low socioeconomic status	Antenatal and postnatal parenting education in infant development from nurse; involvement of family members and friends in child care; linkage of family members with health and human services	"Emergency visit for accidents and poisoning (1st year of life)"	0·12*	0·06*	2·06 (0·83 to 5·15)
			"Emergency visit for accidents and poisoning (2nd year of life)"	0·15*	0·34*	0·40 (0·21 to 0·77)
			"Emergency department visits for injuries/ingestion (25 to 50 months)"	0·47*	0·61*	0·71 (0·49 to 1·04)
an (1983, 'and)	Families predicted to be at risk of child abuse	Postnatal intervention and support from social worker	"Admissions with trauma"	1/103	4/209	0·50 (0·06 to 4·55)
Le (1980, Canada)	Working class families	Postnatal, non-professional emotional and informational support	"Significant falls, cuts, burns, poisonings or other injuries"	1·26**	1·55**	0·73 (0·46 to 1·16)
Gray *et al* (1979, USA)	Families most likely to exhibit abnormal parenting practices	Postnatal emotional support from physician/nurse/lay visitor	"Accidents by maternal report"	16/26	13/25	1·48 (0·49 to 4·5)
Pooled results						0·74 (0·60 to 0·92)

IHDP = infant health and development programme.
*Adjusted mean. **Cumulative accident rate per child.

vention and control groups would almost certainly result in a substantial underestimation of any beneficial effect of home visiting programmes on the occurrence of child abuse, possibly to the extent of reversing the direction of the apparent effect. Indeed, the usefulness of reported abuse as an outcome measure in trials of home visiting deserves reconsideration.

Publication bias is one of the most important potential threats to the validity of systematic reviews. Such bias may arise if certain outcome data are selectively omitted from published reports because the results fail to reach significance. To avoid this type of bias we wrote to the authors of all identified randomised trials of home visiting programmes, asking them to provide any unpublished outcome data on injury or abuse (one further trial was identified by this approach). The authors of nearly half of the studies meeting the first two inclusion criteria, however, could not be traced. These were predominantly small studies and so would make a comparatively minor impact on the overall result. Funnel plots can be used to estimate the extent of publication bias, but because their use is limited to meta-analyses that have enough trials to allow a funnel shape to be visualised, this approach is not helpful in this review.[44]

A recurring issue in the context of systematic reviews is the extent to which the interventions examined are sufficiently comparable for the results from the studies to be combined. The effectiveness of home visiting may depend on its timing, duration, and intensity. Nevertheless, for unintentional childhood injuries no clear heterogeneity was seen in the effect across studies.

IMPLICATIONS

Because most of the trials included in this review used non-professional home visitors, the question of the relative effectiveness of professional versus non-professional home visiting remains unanswered. The observed effect of home visiting on child injury is consistent with a generic effect of home based maternal support. In Britain a programme of home visiting is provided by health visitors. Current health visiting programmes, however, should not be assumed to achieve the effects on childhood injury that are implied by the results of this systematic review. Firstly, the experimental home visiting may have been more intense than that which is typically provided by health visitors. Secondly, in all but one of the trials the intervention was targeted at groups considered to be at increased risk for adverse child health outcomes. This may restrict the extent to which the results are generalisable to programmes of universal health visiting.

The Health of the Nation strategy established child accident prevention as a national priority. Few injury

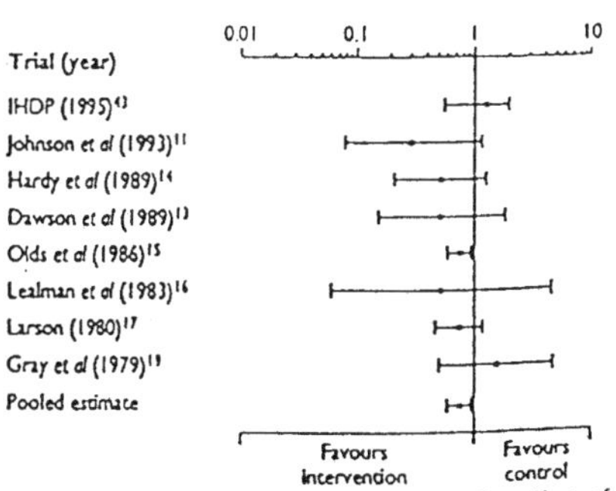

Odds ratios and 95% confidence intervals for effect of home visiting on child injury

Key messages

- The Health of the Nation established prevention of child injury as a national priority
- Home visiting has been proposed as a prevention strategy, but the results from randomised trials are conflicting
- This systematic review of randomised trials shows that home visiting can substantially reduce rates of child injury
- No consistent effect on child abuse was found, but differential surveillance for child abuse between visited groups and control groups is an important weakness in many trials
- The role of health visitors and non-professionals in the prevention of child injury deserves further attention

prevention interventions, however, have been shown to reduce injury rates in randomised controlled trials. Given the results of this systematic review, the effectiveness of home visiting by health visitors and non-professional support agencies in preventing childhood injury deserves further examination.

We thank the authors of the original articles who replied to inquiries and provided data not included in their published articles. We specifically thank Drs Marie McCormick and Pamela Klebanov for conducting new analyses of the data from the infant health and development programme.

Funding: IR was supported by an overseas fellowship from the Health Research Council of New Zealand. SS is a research scholar of the Fonds de la Recherche en Santé in Quebec.

Conflict of interest: None.

Avery JG, Jackson RH. *Children and their accidents*. Edward Arnold: London, 1933.
Kempe CH. Approaches to preventing child abuse: the health visitor concept. *Am J Dis Child* 1976;130:941-2.
3 United States Advisory Board on Child Abuse and Neglect. *Child abuse and neglect: critical first steps in response to a national emergency*. Washington DC: US Government Printing Office, 1990. (Publication no 017-092-00104-5.)
4 Olds DL, Kitzman H. Can home visitation improve the health of women and children at environmental risk? *Pediatrics* 1990;86:108-16.
5 Combs-Orme T, Reis J, Ward LD. Effectiveness of home visits by public health nurses in maternal and child health: an empirical review. *Public Health Rep* 1985;100:490-9.
6 Oxman AD, Cook DJ, Guyatt GH. User's guides to the medical literature. VI. How to use an overview. *JAMA* 1994;272:1367-71.
7 Prendiville W, Elbourne D, Chalmers I. The effects of routine oxytocic administration in the management of the third stage of labor: an overview of the evidence from controlled trials. *Br J Obstet Gynaecol* 1988;95:3-16.
8 Cohen JA. A coefficient of agreement for nominal scales. *Educational and Psychological Measurement* 1960;20:37-46.
9 Wolf B. On estimating the relation between blood group and disease. *Ann Hum Genet* 1965;19:251-3.
10 Marcenko MO, Spence M. Home visitation services for at-risk pregnant and postpartum women: a randomised trial. *Am J Orthopsychiatry* 1994;64:468-78.
11 Johnson Z, Howell F, Molloy B. Community mother's programme: a randomised controlled trial of non-professional intervention in parenting. *BMJ* 1993;306:1449-52.
12 Barth RP. An experimental evaluation of in-home child abuse prevention services. *Child Abuse Negl* 1991;15:363-75.
13 Dawson P, Van Doorninck WJ, Robinson JL. Effects of home based, informal social support on child health. *J Dev Behav Pediatr* 1989;10:63-7.
14 Hardy JB, Streett R. Family support and parenting education in the home: an effective extension of clinic-based preventive health care services for poor children. *J Pediatr* 1989;115:927-31.
15 Olds DL, Henderson CR, Chamberlin R, Tatelbaum R. Preventing child abuse and neglect: a randomised trial of nurse home visitation. *Pediatrics* 1986;78:65-78.
16 Lealman G, Haigh D, Philips J. Predicting and preventing child abuse—an empty hope? *Lancet* 1983;i:1423-4.
17 Larson CP. Efficacy of prenatal and postpartum home visits on child health and development. *Pediatrics* 1980;66:191-7.
18 Siegel E, Bauman KE, Schaefer ES, Saunders MM, Ingram DD. Hospital and home support in infancy: impact on maternal attachment, child abuse and neglect, and health care utilization. *Pediatrics* 1980;66:183-90.
19 Gray JD, Cutler CA, Dean JG, Kempe CH. Prediction and prevention of child abuse and neglect. *Journal of Social Issues* 1979;35:127-39.
20 Infante-Rivard C, Filion G, Baumgarten M, Labelle J, Messier M. A public health home intervention among families of low socioeconomic status. *Children's Health Care* 1989;18:102-7.
21 Casey PH, Kelleher KJ, Bradley RH, Kellogg UW, Kirby RS, Whiteside L. A multifaceted intervention for infants with failure to thrive. *Arch Pediatr Adolesc Med* 1994;148:1071-7.
22 Greenberg RA, Strecher VJ, Bauman KE, Boat BW, Fowler MG, Keyes LL, *et al*. Evaluation of a home-based intervention program to reduce infant passive smoking and lower respiratory illness. *J Behav Med* 1994;17:273-90.

Table 3—*Home visiting and child abuse*

Trial (year, country)	Study population	Intervention	Outcome	Participants visited	Controls	Odds ratio (95% confidence interval)
Marcenko *et al* (1994, USA)	Women at risk of out of home placement of their newborns	Antenatal, postnatal, professional/non-professional to provide peer support; help to identify service needs; home based health education and parenting training	Out of home placement	35/110	15/77	1·93 (0·97 to 3·85)
[illegible]son *et al* ([illegible]993, Republic [illegible]ireland)	Disadvantaged first time mothers	Postnatal, non-professional support and encouragement in child rearing using the child development programme	Abuse unspecified	0/127	3/105	0·11 (0·01 to 2·25)
[illegible]h ([illegible]991, USA)	Parents identified as at risk of engaging in child abuse by community professionals	Antenatal and postnatal, non-professional, informational, emotional, and practical support	Reported abuse	64/97	54/94	1·44 (0·80 to 2·58)
[illegible]ardy *et al* (1989, USA)	Inner city mothers of poor infants	Postnatal, non-professional parenting and childcare education	Suspected abuse	2/131	13/132	0·14 (0·03 to 0·64)
[illegible]awson *et al* (1989, USA)	Pregnant women attending for maternity care not selected for psychosocial risk	Antenatal and postnatal, non-professional emotional support; information and help in using community resources	Reported abuse	5/67	1/44	3·47 (0·39 to 30·74)
[illegible]lds *et al* (1986, USA)	Primiparas who were teenagers, unmarried, or of low socioeconomic status	Antenatal and postnatal parenting education in infant development from nurse; involvement of family members and friends in child care; linkage of family members with health and human services	Registered abuse (age 0-2 years) Registered abuse (age 2-4 years)	0·05* 0·08*	0·10* 0·05*	
[illegible]ealman *et al* (1983, England)	Families predicted to be at risk of child abuse	Postnatal intervention and support from social worker	Registered abuse	1/103	3/209	0·67 (0·07 to 6·55)
[illegible]iegel *et al* (1980, USA)	Women with low income	Postnatal, non-professional support to promote mothers' involvement with their infants and to support mothers in coping with range of stresses	Reported abuse	14/159	9/162	1·64 (0·69 to 3·91)
[illegible]ray *et al* (1979, USA)	Families most likely to exhibit abnormal parenting practices	Postnatal emotional support from physician/nurse/lay	Suspected abuse	0/50	6/50	0·08 (0·00 to 1·52)

*Adjusted means.

23 Currie AL, Gehlbach SH, Massion C, Thompson S. Newborn home visits. *J Fam Pract* 1983;17:635-8.

24 Thompson RJ, Cappleman MW, Conrad HH, Jordan WB. Early intervention program for adolescent mothers and their infants. *J Dev Behav Pediatr* 1982;3:18-21.

25 Yanover MJ, Jones D, Miller MD. Perinatal care of low-risk mothers and infants. *N Engl J Med* 1976;294:702-5.

26 Black MM, Nair P, Kight C, Wachtel R, Roby P, Schler M. Parenting and early development among children of drug abusing mothers: effects of home intervention. *Pediatrics* 1994;94:440-8.

27 Hall LA. Effect of teaching on primiparas' perceptions of their newborn. *Nursing Res* 1980;29:317-21.

28 Lowe ML. Effectiveness of teaching as measured by compliance with medical recommendations. *Nursing Res* 1970;19:59-63.

29 Yauger RA. Does family centered care make a difference? *Nursing Outlook* 1972;20:320-3.

30 Shyne AW, LeMat A, Kogan LS. Evaluating public health nursing service to the maternity patient and her family. *Nursing Outlook* 1963;11:56-8.

31 Stanwick RS, Moffat ME, Robitaille Y, Edmond A, Dok C. An evaluation of the routine public health nurse home visit. *Can J Public Health* 1982; 73:200-5.

32 Field TM, Widmayer SM, Stringer S, Ignatoff E. Teenage, lower class, black mothers and their pre-term infants: an intervention and developmental follow-up. *Child Dev* 1980;51:426-36.

33 Powell C, Grantham-McGregor S. Home visiting of varying frequency and child development. *Pediatrics* 1989;84:157-64.

34 Beckwith L. Intervention with disadvantaged parents of sick pre-term infants. *Psychiatry* 1988;51:242-7.

35 Barnard KE, Magyary D, Sumner G, Booth CL, Mitchell SK, Spieker S. Prevention of parenting alterations for women with low social support. *Psychiatry* 1988;51:248-53.

36 Scarr S, McCartney K. Far from home: an experimental evaluation of the mother-child home program in Bermuda. *Child Dev* 1988;59:531-43.

37 Madden J, O'Hara J, Levenstein P. Home again: effects of the mother-child home program on mother and child. *Child Dev* 1984;55:636-47.

38 Casiro OG, McKenzie ME, McFadyen L, Shapiro C, Seshia MM, MacDonald N, *et al*. Earlier discharge with community base intervention for low birth weight infants: a randomised trial. *Pediatrics* 1993;92:128-34.

39 Vines SW, Williams-Burgess C. Effects of a community health nursing parent-baby (ad)venture program on depression and other selected maternal child health outcomes. *Public Health Nursing* 1994;11:188-95.

40 Johnson DL, Walker T. Primary prevention on behaviour problems in Mexican-American children. *Am J Community Psychol* 1987;15:375-85.

41 Nicol AR, Stretch DD, Davison I, Fundudis T. Controlled comparison of three interventions for mother and toddler problems: preliminary communication. *J R Soc Med* 1984;77:488-91.

42 Olds DL, Kitzman HJ, Cole RE. Effect of home visitation by nurses on caregiving and maternal life course. *Arch Pediatr Adolesc Med* 1995; 149:76.

43 The Infant Health and Development Program. Enhancing the outcomes of low-birth-weight, premature infants. *JAMA* 1990;263:3035-42.

44 Dickersin K, Berlin JA. Meta-analysis: state of the science. *Epidemiol Rev* 1992;143:154-76.

(Accepted 30 November 1995)

Clinical question:

Are the results of this systematic review (systematic review) of therapy valid?

Did the review address a clearly focused question? How likely is it that the search strategy would have missed eligible trials?

Are the inclusion criteria clearly stated?

Are the inclusion criteria relating to population, intervention and comparison groups and outcome appropriate?

How likely is it that the conclusions are valid (i.e. Are the included studies good quality randomised controlled trials)?

If a meta-analysis was performed, were the included studies sufficiently homogeneous to make it appropriate to pool data?

Are the valid results of this systematic review important?

Translating odds ratios to NNTs. The numbers in the body of the table are the NNTs for the corresponding odds ratios at that particular patient's expected event rate (PEER).

		Odds ratios (OR)								
		0.9	0.85	0.8	0.75	0.7	0.65	0.6	0.55	0.5
Patient's event rate (PER)	.05	209[1]	139	104	83	69	59	52	46	41[2]
	.10	110	73	54	43	36	31	27	24	21
	.20	61	40	30	24	20	17	14	13	11
	.30	46	30	22	18	14	12	10	9	8
	.40	40	26	19	15	12	10	9	8	7
	.50[3]	38	25	18	14	11	9	8	7	6
	.70	44	28	20	16	13	10	9	7	6
	.90	101[4]	64	46	34	27	22	18	15	12[5]

[1]The relative risk reduction (RRR) here is 10%.

[2]The RRR here is 49%.

[3]For any OR, NNT is lowest when PEER = .50.

[4]The RRR here is 1%.

[5]The RRR here is 9%.

		Odds ratios (OR)				
		1.1	1.2	1.3	1.4	1.5
Patient's expected event rate (PEER)	.05	212	106	71	54	43
	.10	112	57	38	29	23
	.20	64	33	22	17	14
	.30	49	25	17	13	11
	.40	43	23	16	12	10
	.50[6]	42	22	15	12	10
	.70	51	27	19	15	135
	.90	121	66	47	38	32

The numbers in the body of the table are the NNTs for the corresponding odds ratios at that particular patient's expected event rate (PEER). This table applies both when a good outcome is increased by therapy and when a side-effect is caused by therapy.

Can you apply this valid, important evidence from a systematic review in caring for your patient?

Do these results apply to your patient?

Are my patients so different from those in the review that there are likely to be important differences in treatment effect?

Is the intervention in the studies in the review sufficiently similar to the treatment that I am considering?

Are the outcome measures documented an adequate reflection of the outcomes of importance to my patients?

How great would the potential benefit of therapy actually be for your individual patient?

Method I: In the table on p 1, find the intersection of the closest odds ratio from the overview and the CER that is closest to your patient's expected event rate if they received the control treatment (PEER):

Method II: To calculate the NNT for any OR and PEER:

$$\text{NNT} = \frac{1 - \{\text{PEER} \times (1 - \text{OR})\}}{(1 - \text{PEER}) \times \text{PEER} \times (1 - \text{OR})}$$

Are your patient's values and preferences satisfied by the regimen and its consequences?

Does your patient and you have a clear assessment of their values and preferences?

Are they met by this regimen and its consequences?

Should you believe apparent qualitative differences in the efficacy of therapy in some subgroups of patients? Only if you can say 'yes' to all of the following:

Do they really make biologic and clinical sense?

Is the qualitative difference both clinically (beneficial for some but useless or harmful for others) and statistically significant?

Was this difference hypothesised before the study began (rather than the product of dredging the data), and has it been confirmed in other, independent studies?

Was this one of just a few subgroup analyses carried out in this study?

Additional notes

Clinical question: In children under 5 years, does a health visitor (compared to no health visitor) prevent accidental injury

Are the results of this systematic review (systematic review) of therapy valid?

Did the review address a clearly focused question?	**Yes.**
How likely is it that the search strategy would have missed eligible trials?	**Unlikely to have missed eligible published trials.**
Are the inclusion criteria clearly stated?	**Yes.**
Are the inclusion criteria relating to population, intervention and comparison groups and outcome appropriate?	**Yes. However, criteria includes both intentional and unintentional injury as outcomes, and there is broad mix of populations and interventions.**
How likely is it that the conclusions are valid (i.e. are the included studies good quality randomised controlled trials)?	**Likely. Conclusions not altered by limiting analysis to trials with high quality scores.**
If a meta-analysis was performed, were the included studies sufficiently homogeneous to make it appropriate to pool data?	**Yes for unintentional injury. Heterogeneity noted in studies of intentional injury.**

Are the valid results of this systematic review important?

Translating odds ratios to NNTs. The numbers in the body of the table are the NNTs for the corresponding odds ratios at that particular patient's expected event rate (PEER).

		Odds ratios (OR)								
		0.9	0.85	0.8	0.75	0.7	0.65	0.6	0.55	0.5
Patient's expected event rate (PEER)	.05	209[1]	139	104	83	69	59	52	46	41[2]
	.10	110	73	54	43	36	31	27	24	21
	.20	61	40	30	24	20	17	14	13	11
	.30	46	30	22	18	14	12	10	9	8
	.40	40	26	19	15	12	10	9	8	7
	.50[3]	38	25	18	14	11	9	8	7	6
	.70	44	28	20	16	13	10	9	7	6
	.90	101[4]	64	46	34	27	22	18	15	12[5]

[1]The relative risk reduction (RRR) here is 10%.

[2]The RRR here is 49%.

[3]For any OR, NNT is lowest when PEER = .50.

[4]The RRR here is 1%.

[5]The RRR here is 9%.

		Odds ratios (OR)				
		1.1	1.2	1.3	1.4	1.5
	.05	212	106	71	54	43
Patient's	.10	112	57	38	29	23
expected	.20	64	33	22	17	14
event	.30	49	25	17	13	11
rate	.40	43	23	16	12	10
(PEER)	.50[6]	42	22	15	12	10
	.70	51	27	19	15	135
	.90	121	66	47	38	32

The numbers in the body of the table are the NNTs for the corresponding odds ratios at that particular patient's expected event rate (PEER). This table applies both when a good outcome is increased by therapy and when a side-effect is caused by therapy.

Results: For unintentional injuries, pooled odds ratio is <1 which favours intervention; i.e. there are fewer unintentional injuries in children whose mother was visited at home than in those not visited.

Pooled OR = 0.74 with 95% CI of 0.6 to 0.92. As CI does not include 1, result is statistically significant.

Can you apply this valid, important evidence from a systematic review in caring for your patient?

Do these results apply to your patient?

Are my patients so different from those in the review that there are likely to be important differences in treatment effect?	**Maybe. Studies mainly involved 'high-risk' families.**
Is the intervention in the studies in the review sufficiently similar to the treatment that I am considering?	**Maybe. Most studies involved non-professional visitors.**
Are the outcome measures documented an adequate reflection of the outcomes of importance to my patients?	**Yes.**

How great would the potential benefit of therapy actually be for your individual patient?

Method 1: In the table on p 1, find the intersection of the closest odds ratio from the overview and the CER that is closest to your patient's expected event rate if they received the control treatment (PEER):	**OR = 0.74** **Assume PEER for injuries is only 5%** **NNT = 83**
Method II: To calculate the NNT for any OR and PEER: $NNT = \frac{1 - \{PEER \times (1 - OR)\}}{(1 - PEER) \times PEER \times (1 - OR)}$	**Your PEER is 0.05, so with OR of 0.74, NNT = 80**

Are your patient's values and preferences satisfied by the regimen and its consequences?

Do your patient and you have a clear assessment of their values and preferences?	**Yes.**
Are they met by this regimen and its consequences?	**Not entirely. Need information on intensity of visiting and effect and acceptability of professional compared with non-professional visitors.**

Should you believe apparent qualitative differences in the efficacy of therapy in some subgroups of patients? Only if you can say 'yes' to all of the following:

Do they really make biologic and clinical sense?	**Yes, unintentional injuries are different from intentional injuries.**
Is the qualitative difference both clinically (beneficial for some but useless or harmful for others) and statistically significant?	**Yes.**
Was this difference hypothesised before the study began (rather than the product of dredging the data), and has it been confirmed in other, independent studies?	**Yes.**
Was this one of just a few subgroup analyses carried out in this study?	**Yes.**

Additional notes

1 Despite the ill-defined intervention (i.e. professional and non-professional visitors) and the crude outcome measures (some parent recall, some hospital attendance) there is a statistically significant result which suggests that home visiting has a real impact on children's unintentional injuries.
2 When outcome is rare, the relative risk and odds ratio approximate.

CHILDHOOD INJURIES – REDUCED BY HOME VISITS

Appraised by O Duperrex and R Gilbert: 3 March 1999
Expiry date: March 2000.

Clinical Bottom Line
Home visiting can reduce the number of unintentional injuries.

Citation
Roberts I, Kramer MS, and Suissa S (1996) Does home visiting prevent childhood injury? *BMJ* **312:** 29–33.

Clinical Question
In children, can home visiting reduce the injury rate?

Search Terms
'home visiting' and 'child' and 'injury' and 'randomised-controlled-trial'.

The Study
Systematic review of 11 RCTs including 3433 participants.

The Evidence
Pooled OR of home visiting Vs 'control' for unintentional injuries is 0.74 (95% CI 0.6–0.92).

If baseline risk for unintentional injuries is 5%, NNT is 80.

If baseline risk for unintentional injuries is 15%, NNT is 29.

Comments
1 The populations in all trials were disadvantaged.
2 Interventions varied: visits were by non-professionals and occurred during and/or after pregnancy and at different intensities.
3 Outcomes varied from hospital attendance to parent recall of injuries.
4 The review on intentional injuries is difficult to interpret as reporting of injuries was confounded by increased detection in the home visiting groups.

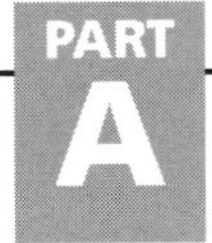

Critical appraisal of a systematic review

EBCH SESSION

4

SECTION 2

Systematic reviews and searching the primary literature

Section 2: Albumin for critically ill patients

The Drugs and Therapeutics Committee of your hospital (a DGH) is reviewing the use of human albumin solution in the hospital. The paediatric department is approached because of its use of human albumin solution. You explain that the main use is in children with meningococcal sepsis in whom there is a high mortality. You are asked to consider the use of crystalloids in these patients because it is cheaper and there is not the theoretical risk of transmission of infection as there is with albumin (a blood product). Furthermore, the committee is concerned about recent publicity citing increased mortality in patients given albumin.

What policy do you recommend for children with septic shock? You pose the question, in children with meningococcal septicaemia who are critically ill, does albumin decrease the risk of mortality compared with crystalloid solution?

Search strategy for albumin

Type in:
1 ALBUMIN in TI,AB,MESH
2 explode "Serum-Albumin" / all subheadings
3 #1 or #2
4 child*
5 #3 and #4
6 DEATH in TI,AB,MESH
7 #5 and #6
8 PT = "META-ANALYSIS"
9 #7 and #8

Using this strategy, you find the enclosed Cochrane Review (*BMJ* 1998; **317:** 235–40).

Read the systematic review and decide:
1 Is the evidence from this systematic review valid?
2 Is this valid evidence from this systematic review important?
3 Can you apply this valid and important evidence from this systematic review in caring for your patient?

If you want to read some strategies for answering these sorts of questions, you could have a look at pp 97–9, 140–41 and 166–72 in *Evidence-based Medicine*.

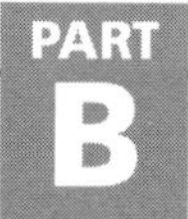

Searching for evidence in the primary literature

Colleagues from the library will come and whet your appetite for learning how to search for evidence in the clinical literature or hone the searching skills you already have developed. So bring along the clinical questions you generated in Session 2 (or any that you have generated in the meantime). Efficient EBM searching strategies that trade-off the sensitivity and specificity of your searches are on the next page.

If you haven't already done your search for your presentation in Sessions 6 and 7, now would be a good time to do it!

BEST SINGLE TERMS AND COMBINATIONS FOR HIGH SENSITIVITY MEDLINE SEARCHES ON THE BEST STUDIES OF TREATMENT, DIAGNOSIS, PROGNOSIS, OR CAUSE.

Search strategy	Sensitivity[1]	Specificity	Precision
For studies of treatment:			
Clinical trial (pt)	0.93	0.92	0.49
Randomised controlled trial (pt) or Drug therapy (sh) or Therapeutic use (sh) or Random: (tw)	0.99	0.74	0.22
For studies of prognosis:			
Exp cohort studies	0.60	0.80	0.11
Incidence or Exp mortality or Follow up studies or Mortality: (sh) or Prognosis: (tw) or Predict: (tw) or Course (tw)	0.92	0.73	0.11
For studies of aetiology or cause:			
Risk (tw)	0.67	0.79	0.15
Exp cohort studies or Exp risk or Odds and ratio: (tw) or Relative and risk: (tw) or Case and control: (tw)	0.82	0.70	0.14
For studies of diagnosis:			
Diagnosis (pe)	0.80	0.77	0.09
Exp Sensitivity and specificity or Diagnosis: (pe) or Diagnostic use or Sensitivity: (tw) or Specificity: (tw)	0.92	0.73	0.09

[1]**Sensitivity**, as defined in the study on which the table is based, is the proportion of studies in MEDLINE meeting criteria for scientific soundness and clinical relevance that are detected. **Specificity** is the proportion of less sound/relevant studies that are excluded by the search strategy. **Precision** is the proportion of all citations retrieved that are both sound and relevant (source: *Evidence-based Medicine*; see also the Web pages).

Papers

Human albumin administration in critically ill patients: systematic review of randomised controlled trials

Cochrane Injuries Group Albumin Reviewers

Abstract

Objective: To quantify effect on mortality of administering human albumin or plasma protein fraction during management of critically ill patients.
Design: Systematic review of randomised controlled trials comparing administration of albumin or plasma protein fraction with no administration or with administration of crystalloid solution in critically ill patients with hypovolaemia, burns, or hypoalbuminaemia.
Subjects: 30 randomised controlled trials including 1419 randomised patients.
Main outcome measure: Mortality from all causes at end of follow up for each trial.
Results: For each patient category the risk of death in the albumin treated group was higher than in the comparison group. For hypovolaemia the relative risk of death after albumin administration was 1.46 (95% confidence interval 0.97 to 2.22), for burns the relative risk was 2.40 (1.11 to 5.19), and for hypoalbuminaemia it was 1.69 (1.07 to 2.67). Pooled relative risk of death with albumin administration was 1.68 (1.26 to 2.23). Pooled difference in the risk of death with albumin was 6% (95% confidence interval 3% to 9%) with a fixed effects model. These data suggest that for every 17 critically ill patients treated with albumin there is one additional death.
Conclusions: There is no evidence that albumin administration reduces mortality in critically ill patients with hypovolaemia, burns, or hypoalbuminaemia and a strong suggestion that it may increase mortality. These data suggest that use of human albumin in critically ill patients should be urgently reviewed and that it should not be used outside the context of rigorously conducted, randomised controlled trials.

Introduction

In patients with acute and chronic illness serum albumin concentration is inversely related to risk of death. A systematic review of cohort studies meeting specified criteria estimated that for each 2.5 g/l decrement in serum albumin concentration the risk of death increases by between 24% and 56%.[1] The association persists after adjustment for other known risk factors and pre-existing illness, and some commentators have suggested the possibility of the albumin molecule having a direct protective effect.[1] Partly as a result of the association between serum albumin and mortality, human albumin solutions are now used in the management of a diverse range of medical and surgical problems. Licensed indications for human albumin solution are the emergency treatment of shock and other conditions in which restoration of blood volume is urgent, the acute management of burns, and clinical situations associated with hypoproteinaemia.[2]

Compared with other colloidal solutions and with crystalloid solutions, human albumin solutions are expensive.[3] Volume for volume, human albumin solution is twice as expensive as hydroxyethyl starch and over 30 times more expensive than crystalloid solutions such as sodium chloride or Ringer's lactate. Because of the high cost and limited availability of human albumin, it is imperative that its use should be restricted to the indications for which it has been shown to be effective. To quantify the effect on mortality of human albumin solution in the management of critically ill patients with hypovolaemia from injury or surgery, burns, and hypoproteinaemia, we conducted a systematic review of randomised controlled trials.

Methods

Identification of trials

Our aim was to identify all relevant randomised controlled trials that were available for review by March 1998. A randomised controlled trial was defined as a trial in which the subjects followed were assigned prospectively to one of two (or more) interventions by random allocation or some quasi-random method of allocation. This definition was agreed at an international meeting held in Oxford in November 1992 in association with the official opening of the UK Cochrane Centre. We sought to identify all randomised controlled trials of administration of human albumin or plasma protein fraction (supplemental albumin or plasma protein fraction compared with no albumin or plasma protein fraction or with a crystalloid solution) in critically ill patients with hypovolaemia from trauma or surgery, with burns, or with hypoalbuminaemia. Studies that compared different levels of albumin supplementation were also included.

Editorial by Offringa and *Letters* p 277

Cochrane Injuries Group, Department of Epidemiology and Public Health, Institute of Child Health, London WC1N 1EH
Ian Roberts, *director, child health monitoring unit*
Ian.Roberts@ich.ucl.ac.uk

BMJ 1998;317:235–40

Trials were identified by computerised searches of the Cochrane Controlled Trials Register, Medline, Embase, and BIDS Index to Scientific and Technical Proceedings (search strategies are available from IR); by hand searching 29 international journals and the proceedings of several international meetings on fluid resuscitation; by checking the reference lists of all included trials; and by contacting the authors of identified trials and asking them about any other published or unpublished trials that may have been conducted. There were no language restrictions. To identify unpublished trials we searched the register of the Medical Editors' Trial Amnesty,[4] and contacted the Medical Directors of Bio Products Laboratory (Zenalb), Centeon (Albuminar), and Alpha Therapeutic UK (Albutein).

Outcome measures and data extraction

The outcome measure was mortality from all causes at the end of the follow up period scheduled for each trial. For all trials we collected data on the type of participants, details about the interventions, the quality of concealment of allocation, and mortality at the end of follow up. We rated quality of allocation concealment using the method proposed by Schulz et al.[5] We sought mortality data in simple categorical form, and we did

Summary of randomised trials comparing albumin with no albumin or crystalloid that met criteria for inclusion

Trial	Critical illness	No of patients	Intervention	Control	Length of follow up	Total No of deaths	Allocation concealment*
Hypovolaemia							
Skillman et al[31]	Surgery	16	25% concentrated salt-poor albumin 1 g/kg and 5% albumin in saline	Ringer's lactate with 5% dextrose	1 day	Not known	2
Shah et al[27]	Trauma	20	5% salt-poor albumin in Ringer's lactate	Ringer's lactate	Unspecified	5	3
Lowe et al[20]	Trauma	171	50 g albumin/200 ml Ringer's lactate	Ringer's lactate	5 days	6	3
Boutros et al[9]	Surgery	24	Albumin in 5% dextrose	5% dextrose in lactated Ringer's (n=9) 5% dextrose in 0.45% NaCl (n=8)	4 days	2	2
Virgilio et al[33]	Surgery	29	5% albumin in Ringer's lactate	Ringer's lactate	2½ weeks	2	2
Lucas et al[21]	Trauma	52	150 g salt-poor albumin during operation, 150 g/day for 5 days postoperatively	No albumin	To positive fluid balance or oral intake	7	1
Zetterstrom et al[37]	Surgery	30	20% albumin 100 ml at end of operation, 200 ml on day of operation, 100 ml/day for next 3 days	No albumin	Unspecified	1	3
Zetterstrom[38]	Surgery	18	5% albumin to keep pulmonary arterial occlusion pressure equal to preoperative level	Balanced electrolyte solution of Ringer's type to keep pulmonary arterial pressure equal to preoperative level	Unspecified	2	3
Grundman et al[17]	Surgery	17	Human albumin and crystalloid	Crystalloid only	5 days	1	2
Rackow et al[30]	Trauma and sepsis	17	5% albumin	0.9% NaCl	To discharge	12	2
Gallagher et al[12]	Surgery	10	5% albumin	Ringer's lactate	1 day	0	3
Nielsen et al[23]	Surgery	26	80 g albumin in units of 100 ml 20% albumin on day of operation, 20 g daily for next 3 days	No albumin	4 days	0	2
Prien et al[26]	Surgery	12	20% albumin to maintain central venous pressure at preoperative level	Ringer's lactate	Unspecified	0	2
Boldt et al[8]	Surgery	30	5% albumin	No albumin	1 day	0	3
McNulty et al[22]	Surgery	28	5% albumin	Isotonic crystalloid	Unspecified	Not known	2
Woods et al[36]	Surgery	69	Albumin supplementation	No supplementation	To discharge	1	1
Pockaj et al[25]	Vascular leak syndrome	107	5% albumin in 0.9% NaCl	0.9% NaCl	Unspecified	0	2
Tølløfsrud et al[32]	Surgery	20	4% albumin when fluid required	Ringer's acetate	48 hours	1	3
So et al[28]	Hypotensive preterm infant	63	5% albumin 10 ml/kg over 30 minutes	0.9% NaCl 10 ml/kg over 30 minutes	To discharge	12	3
Woittiez et al[34]	Surgery	31	20% albumin	0.9% NaCl	Unspecified	12	3
Burns							
Jelenko et al[18]	Burns	14	Hypertonic crystalloid with 12.5 g/l albumin	Ringer's lactate	5 days	3	2
Goodwin et al[14]	Burns	79	2.5% albumin in Ringer's lactate	Ringer's lactate	To discharge	14	2
Greenhalgh et al[15]	Burns	70	25% albumin to maintain serum levels between 2.5 and 3.5 g/dl	No albumin unless levels dropped below 1.5 g/dl	To discharge	10	3
Hypoproteinaemia							
Bland et al[7]	Hypoproteinaemia	27	25% albumin 8 ml/kg	5% glucose 8 ml/kg	Unspecified	5	2
Nilsson et al[24]	Hypoalbuminaemia (postoperative)	59	20-25 g albumin/day for 3 days starting day after operation	No supplemental albumin	To discharge	1	3
Brown et al[10]	Hypoalbuminaemia	67	TPN with added albumin	No supplemental albumin	To discharge	10	1
Foley et al[11]	Hypoalbuminaemia	40	TPN with added albumin (25-50 g/day 25% albumin)	No supplemental albumin	To discharge	13	1
Kanarek et al[19]	Hypoalbuminaemia	24	TPN with added albumin	No supplemental albumin	Unspecified	5	3
Wojtysiak et al[35]	Hypoalbuminaemia	30	TPN with added albumin	No supplemental albumin	5 days	0	1
Greenough et al[16]	Hypoalbuminaemic sick preterm infants	40	20% salt-poor albumin 5 ml/kg with maintenance fluids	5 ml/kg maintenance fluid placebo	24 hours after infusion	10	3
Golub et al[13]	Hypoalbuminaemia	219	37.5 g/day albumin until serum albumin >3.0 g/dl	No supplemental albumin	To discharge	18	3
Rubin et al[29]	Hypoalbuminaemia	36	TPN with added albumin	No supplemental albumin	To discharge	3	3

TPN=Total parenteral nutrition. *Allocation concealment: 1=inadequate, 2=unclear, 3=adequate.

not extract data on time to death. If a report did not include the numbers of deaths in each group, we sought these data from the authors. Two reviewers independently extracted the data, and any disagreements were resolved by discussion.

Data analysis and statistical methods

We used the Mantel-Haenszel method to calculate relative risks, risk differences, and 95% confidence intervals for death for each trial on an intention to treat basis using RevMan (Review Manager) statistical software. When there are no events in one group the software adds 0.5 to each cell of the 2×2 table. We tested heterogeneity between trials using χ^2 tests, with $P \leq 0.05$ indicating significant heterogeneity. As long as statistical heterogeneity did not exist, we used a fixed effects model to calculate summary relative risks and 95% confidence intervals.

To examine the extent to which the results of the meta-analyses may have been biased as a result of the selective inclusion of randomised trials with positive findings (publication and other selection bias), we prepared a funnel plot and used the regression approach to assessing funnel plot asymmetry proposed by Egger et al.[6] We used the log odds ratio in the funnel plot because this is the measure that is used in the regression test of funnel plot asymmetry as described by Egger et al. Using simple unweighted linear regression, we regressed the standard normal deviate (defined as the log odds ratio divided by its standard error) against the estimate's precision (defined as the inverse of the standard error). The larger the deviation of the intercept of the regression line from zero, the greater the asymmetry and the more likely it is that the meta-analysis will yield biased estimates of effect. As suggested by Egger et al, we considered $P < 0.1$ to indicate significant asymmetry.

Results

We identified a total of 32 randomised controlled trials that met the study's inclusion criteria.[7-38] The table shows details of these trials. Mortality data were available either from the published report or on contact with the authors in 30 of these trials. The two trials for which mortality data could not be obtained included a total of 42 randomised patients, comprising 3% of the total number of randomised patients in all trials meeting our inclusion criteria.[22 31] One of the trials was an unpublished trial registered in the Medical Editors' Trial Amnesty, and we obtained further details, including data on mortality, directly from the trialist. In six trials there were no deaths in either the intervention or comparison groups.[8 12 23 25 26 35]

The trial by Lucas et al was reported in five publications.[21 39-42] An early report gave the mortality data for 52 randomised patients, 27 allocated to receive albumin and 25 allocated to receive no albumin.[21] Subsequent publications indicated that recruitment to the trial continued until 94 patients were randomised. Mortality data for all the 94 patients were not published, nor were they available on contact with the author. Consequently, we present the outcome data for the 52 patients.

Of the 24 trials in which one or more deaths occurred in either the intervention or control groups,

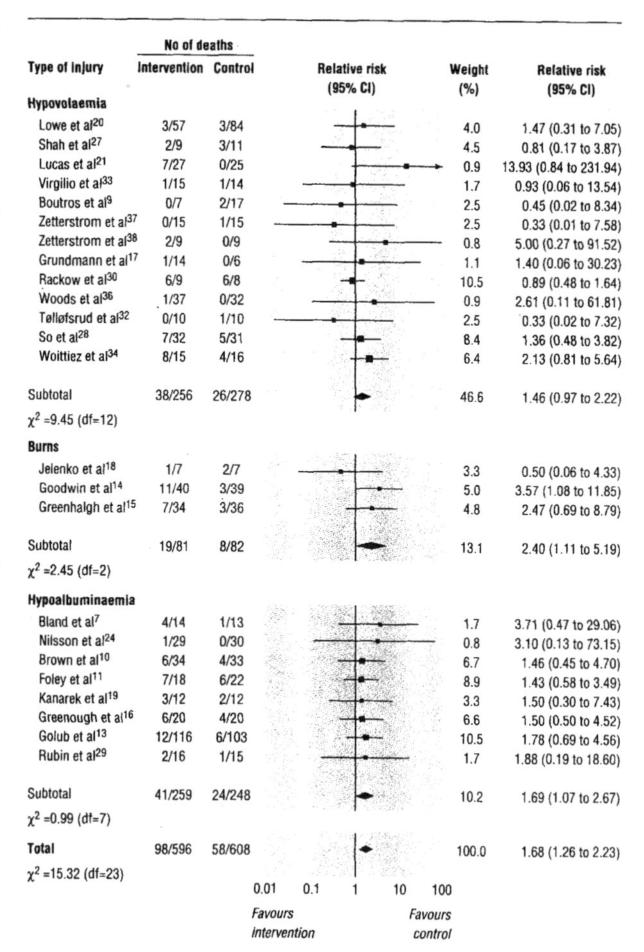

Fig 1 Fixed effects model of relative risks (95% confidence interval) of death associated with intervention (fluid resuscitation with albumin or plasma protein fraction) compared with control (no albumin or plasma protein fraction or resuscitation with a crystalloid solution) in critically ill patients

13 included a method of allocation concealment that would be expected to reduce the risk of foreknowledge of treatment allocation (pharmacy controlled randomisation or serially numbered sealed opaque envelopes). In seven trials this was unclear, and in four trials concealment was inadequate (table).

In each of the patient categories the risk of death in the albumin treated group was higher than in the comparison group (fig 1). For hypovolaemia the relative risk of death after albumin administration was 1.46 (95% confidence interval 0.97 to 2.22), for burns the relative risk was 2.40 (1.11 to 5.19), and for hypoalbuminaemia the it was 1.69 (1.07 to 2.67). There was no significant heterogeneity either between or within the groups of trials, or overall ($\chi^2 = 15.32$, df=23, $P > 0.2$). The pooled relative risk of death with albumin administration was 1.68 (1.26 to 2.23).

There was no significant heterogeneity in the risk difference for mortality ($\chi^2 = 36.69$, df=29, $P > 0.1$). The pooled difference in the risk of death with albumin was 6% (95% confidence interval 3% to 9%).

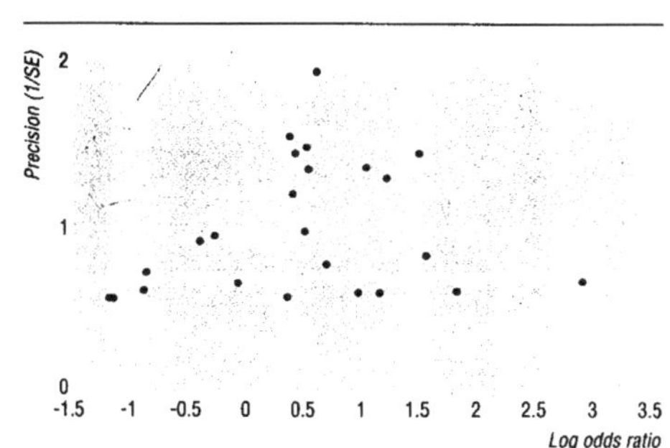

Fig 2 Funnel plot for the 24 trials in which deaths occurred and that were used in systematic review

Figure 2 shows a funnel plot for the 24 trials in which deaths occurred. There was no clear evidence of asymmetry, and the regression approach to funnel plot asymmetry yielded an intercept of −0.39 and P = 0.33, indicating no statistical evidence of selection bias.

We repeated the analyses for the 13 trials with deaths in which allocation concealment was adequate.[13 15 16 19 20 24 27-29 32 34 37 38] For hypovolaemia the relative risk of death with albumin administration was 1.39 (0.80 to 2.40), for burns the relative risk was 2.47 (0.69 to 8.79), and for hypoalbuminaemia it was 1.71 (0.92 to 3.18). There was no substantial heterogeneity between the trials in the various categories ($\chi^2 = 4.42$, df = 12, $P > 0.2$), and the pooled relative risk of death with albumin administration was 1.61 (1.09 to 2.38). Thus, restricting the analyses to the adequately concealed trials had almost no effect on the relative risks in each group or overall.

Discussion

We found no evidence that albumin reduced mortality and a strong suggestion that it might increase the risk of death in patients with hypovolaemia, burns, or hypoproteinaemia. Overall, the risk of death in patients treated with albumin was 6% (95% confidence interval 3% to 9%) higher than in patients not given albumin.

Limitations of study

Mortality was selected as the outcome measure in this systematic review for several reasons. In the context of critical illness, death or survival is a clinically relevant outcome that is of immediate importance to patients, and data on death are reported in nearly all studies. Furthermore, one might expect that mortality data would be less prone to measurement error or biased reporting than would data on pathophysiological outcomes. The use of a pathophysiological end point as a surrogate for an adverse outcome assumes a direct relationship between the two, an assumption that may sometimes be inappropriate. Finally, when trials collect data on a number of physiological end points, there is the potential for bias due to the selective publication of end points showing striking treatment effects. Because we obtained mortality data for all but two of the included trials, the likelihood of bias due to selective publication of trial outcomes is minimal. We examined mortality from all causes because the attribution of cause of death in critically ill patients, many of whom may have multiorgan failure, can be problematic and may be prone to bias. Length of follow up was not specified in many of the trials, but when these data were available, follow up was for the first week or until hospital discharge.

Although publication bias is a potent threat to the validity of systematic reviews, it is unlikely to have had an important impact in this study. There was no evidence of funnel plot asymmetry on visual inspection, and there was no statistical evidence of asymmetry from linear regression analysis.

In some of the trials included in this review allocation concealment was inadequate or unclear. As a result, it is possible that more severely ill patients were preferentially allocated to albumin treated groups, which could account for the increased mortality in these groups. Nevertheless, when we repeated the analyses for only those trials in which the method of allocation concealment would be expected to reduce the risk of foreknowledge of allocation, the point estimates were almost identical.

Implications of results

To what extent are the results of this review of 30 relatively small randomised trials of albumin administration generalisable to clinical practice? We believe that this is a matter for judgment by the responsible clinician faced with an individual patient.[43] However, the advantage of an overview such as ours is that, since it includes many studies, the results are based on a wide range of patients. Because the results were consistent across the studies, they might reasonably be taken to apply to this wide variety of patients.[43] Moreover, the evidence that we have brought together is, as far as we can ensure, the totality of the available randomised evidence for the use of albumin in hypovolaemia, burns, and hypoalbuminaemia, the indications for which albumin is currently licensed.

Is there a plausible mechanism by which human albumin might increase mortality? Albumin is used in hypovolaemia and hypoalbuminaemia because it is believed to be effective in replacing volume and supporting colloid oncotic pressure.[44] However, albumin is also believed to have anticoagulant properties, inhibiting platelet aggregation and enhancing the inhibition of factor Xa by antithrombin III.[44] Such anticoagulant activity might be detrimental in critically ill patients, particularly those with haemorrhagic hypovolaemia. Furthermore, albumin has been shown to distribute across the capillary membrane, a process that is accelerated in critically ill patients.[45] It has been suggested that increased leakage of albumin into the extravascular spaces might reduce the oncotic pressure difference across the capillary wall, making oedema more likely.[45]

Conclusions

Because this review was based on relatively small trials in which there were only a small number of deaths the results must be interpreted with caution. Nevertheless, we believe that a reasonable conclusion from these results is that the use of human albumin in the management of critically ill patients should be reviewed. A strong argument could be made that human albumin should not be used outside the context of a properly concealed and otherwise rigorously conducted randomised controlled trial with

Key messages

- Human albumin solution has been used in the treatment of critically ill patients for over 50 years
- Currently, the licensed indications for use of albumin are emergency treatment of shock, acute management of burns, and clinical situations associated with hypoproteinaemia
- Our systematic review of randomised controlled trials showed that, for each of these patient categories, the risk of death in the albumin treated group was higher than in the comparison group
- The pooled relative risk of death with albumin was 1.68 (95% confidence interval 1.26 to 2.23) and the pooled difference in the risk of death was 6% (3% to 9%) or six additional deaths for every 100 patients treated
- We consider that use of human albumin solution in critically ill patients should be urgently reviewed

mortality as the end point. Until such data become available, there is also a case for a review of the licensed indications for albumin use.

This review will also be published in the *Cochrane Library*, where it will be regularly updated to take account of new data and comments on this version.

We thank the Intensive Care National Audit and Research Centre in London for help with identifying trials for this review and for their extensive hand searching. We thank A J Woittiez for providing unpublished trial data from the trial that was registered in the Medical Editors' Trial Amnesty. We thank Elizabeth Bryant, information officer at Centeon, and Martin O'Fobve, at Bio Products, for searching their databases for albumin trials. We thank Anne Greenough for re-examining individual patient records in order to provide data on mortality. We thank Iain Chalmers, Jos Kleijnen, Richard Peto, Dave Signorini, and David Yates for their comments on the manuscript.

Contributors (listed alphabetically): Phil Alderson (UK Cochrane Centre) searched The Cochrane Controlled Trials Register for relevant trials, extracted the data from the trials, and commented on the paper. Frances Bunn (Institute of Child Health) searched the Cochrane Injuries Group Specialised Register for relevant trials, obtained copies of relevant papers, wrote to authors for further information on allocation concealment, and commented on the paper. Carol Lefebvre (UK Cochrane Centre) designed the search strategies for The Cochrane Controlled Trials Register and Embase, and searched these two databases for relevant trials. Leah Li (Institute of Child Health) did the funnel plot and the regression test of funnel plot asymmetry. Alain Li Wan Po (Centre for Evidence-Based Pharmacotherapy, University of Nottingham) helped to write the paper. Ian Roberts (Institute of Child Health) designed the protocol, extracted data from the trials, contacted authors for unpublished data, and wrote the paper. Gillian Schierhout proposed the study hypothesis and conducted preliminary searches of Medline, Embase, and BIDS Index to Scientific and Technical Proceedings.

Funding: The infrastructure of the Cochrane Injuries Group is supported by the NHS Research and Development Programme.

Conflict of interest: None.

1 Goldwasser P, Feldman J. Association of serum albumin and mortality risk. *J Clin Epidemiol* 1997;50:693-703.
2 *ABPI compendium of data sheets and summaries of product characteristics 1998-99*. London: Association of the British Pharmaceutical Industries, 1998.
3 McClelland DB. Human albumin solutions. *BMJ* 1990;300:35-7.
4 Medical Editors' Trial Amnesty, The Cochrane Controlled Trials Register. In: *The Cochrane Library*. Oxford: Update Software, 1998. Updated quarterly.
5 Schulz KF, Chalmers I, Hayes RJ, Altman DG. Dimensions of methodological quality associated with estimates of treatment effects in controlled trials. *JAMA* 1995;273:408-12.
6 Egger M, Davey Smith G, Schneider M, Minder C. Bias in meta-analyses detected by a simple graphical test. *BMJ* 1997;315:629-34.
7 Bland RD, Clarke TL, Harden LB. Rapid infusion of sodium bicarbonate and albumin into high-risk premature infants soon after birth: a controlled, prospective trial. *Am J Obstet Gynecol* 1976;124:263-7.
8 Boldt J, Knothe C, Zickmann B, Andres P, Dapper F, Hempelmann G. Influence of different intravascular volume therapies on platelet function in patients undergoing cardiopulmonary bypass. *Anesth Analg* 1993;76:1185-90.
9 Boutros AR, Ruess R, Olson L, Hoyt JL, Baker WH. Comparison of hemodynamic, pulmonary, and renal effects of use of three types of fluids after major surgical procedures on the abdominal aorta. *Crit Care Med* 1979;7:9-13.
10 Brown RO, Bradley JE, Bekemeyer WB, Luther RW. Effect of albumin supplementation during parenteral nutrition on hospital morbidity. *Crit Care Med* 1988;16:1177-82.
11 Foley EF, Borlase BC, Dzik WH, Bistrian BR, Benotti PN. Albumin supplementation in the critically ill: a prospective randomised trial. *Arch Surg* 1990;125:739-42.
12 Gallagher JD, Moore RA, Kerns D, Jose AB, Botros SB, Flicker S, et al. Effects of colloid or crystalloid administration on pulmonary extravascular water in the postoperative period after coronary artery bypass grafting. *Anesth Analg* 1985;64:753-8.
13 Golub R, Sorrento JJ Jr, Cantu R Jr, Nierman DM, Moideen A, Stein HD. Efficacy of albumin supplementation in the surgical intensive care unit: a prospective, randomized study. *Crit Care Med* 1994;22:613-9.
14 Goodwin CW, Dorethy J, Lam V, Pruitt BA Jr. Randomized trial of efficacy of crystalloid and colloid resuscitation on hemodynamic response and lung water following thermal injury. *Ann Surg* 1983;197:520-31.
15 Greenhalgh DG, Housinger TA, Kagan RJ, Rieman M, James L, Novak S, et al. Maintenance of serum albumin levels in paediatric burn patients: a prospective, randomized trial [with discussion]. *J Trauma* 1995;39:67-73. (Discussion 1995;39:73-4.)
16 Greenough A, Emery E, Hird MF, Gamsu HR. Randomised controlled trial of albumin infusion in ill pre-term infants. *Eur J Pediatr* 1993;152:157-9.
17 Grundmann R, Meyer H. The significance of colloid osmotic pressure measurement after crystalloid and colloid infusions. *Intensive Care Med* 1982;8:179-86.
18 Jelenko C 3rd, Williams JB, Wheeler ML, Callaway BD, Fackler VK, Albers CA, et al. Studies in shock and resuscitation. I: Use of a hypertonic, albumin-containing, fluid demand regimen (HALFD) in resuscitation. *Crit Care Med* 1979;7:157-67.
19 Kanarek KS, Williams PR, Blair C. Concurrent administration of albumin with total parenteral nutrition in sick new-born infants. *J Parenter Enteral Nutr* 1992;16:49-53.
20 Lowe RJ, Moss GS, Jilek J, Levine HD. Crystalloid vs colloid in the aetiology of pulmonary failure after trauma: a randomized trial in man. *Surgery* 1977;1:676-83.
21 Lucas CE, Weaver D, Higgins RF, Ledgerwood AM, Johnson SD, Bouwman DL. Effects of albumin versus non-albumin resuscitation on plasma volume and renal excretory function. *J Trauma* 1978;18:565-70.
22 McNulty SE, Sharkey SJ, Asam B, Lee JH. Evaluation of STAT-CRIT hematocrit determination in comparison to coulter and centrifuge: the effects of isotonic hemodilution and albumin administration. *Anesth Analg* 1993;76:830-4.
23 Nielsen OM, Engell HC. Extra-cellular fluid volume and distribution in relation to changes in plasma colloid osmotic pressure after major surgery. A randomised study. *Acta Chir Scand* 1985;151:221-5.
24 Nilsson E, Lamke O, Liljedahl SO, Elfstrom K. Is albumin therapy worthwhile in surgery for colorectal cancer? *Acta Chir Scand* 1980;146:619-22.
25 Pockaj BA, Yang JC, Lotze MT, Lange JR, Spencer WF, Steinberg S, et al. A prospective randomized trial evaluating colloid versus crystalloid resuscitation in the treatment of the vascular leak syndrome associated with interleukin-2 therapy. *J Immunother* 1994;15:22-8.
26 Prien T, Backhaus N, Pelster F, Pircher W, Bunte H, Lawin P. Effect of intraoperative fluid administration and colloid osmotic pressure on the formation of intestinal edema during gastrointestinal surgery. *J Clin Anesth* 1990;2:317-23.
27 Shah DM, Browner BD, Dutton RE, Newell JC, Powers SR. Cardiac output and pulmonary wedge pressure. *Arch Surg* 1977;112:1161-4.
28 So KW, Fok TF, Ng PC, Wong WW, Cheung KL. Randomised controlled trial of colloid or crystalloid in hypotensive pre-term infants. *Arch Dis Child* 1997;76:F43-6.
29 Rubin H, Carlson S, DeMeo M, Ganger D, Craig R. Randomized, double-blind study of intravenous human albumin in hypoalbuminaemic patients receiving total parenteral nutrition. *Crit Care Med* 1997;25:249-52.
30 Rackow EC, Falk JL, Fein IA, Siegel JS, Packman MI, Haupt MT, et al. Fluid resuscitation in circulatory shock: a comparison of the cardiorespiratory effects of albumin, hetastarch, and saline solutions in patients with hypovolemic and septic shock. *Crit Care Med* 1983;11:839-50.
31 Skillman JJ, Restall DS, Salzman EW. Randomized trial of albumin vs. electrolyte solutions during abdominal aortic operations. *Surgery* 1975;78:291-303.
32 Tølløfsrud S, Svennevig JL, Breivik H, Kongsgaard U, Øzer M, Hysing E, et al. Fluid balance and pulmonary functions during and after coronary artery bypass surgery: Ringer's acetate compared with dextran, polygeline, or albumin. *Acta Anaesthesiol Scand* 1995;39:671-7.
33 Virgilio RW, Rice CL, Smith DE, James OR, Zarins CK, Hobelmann CF, et al. Crystalloid vs. colloid resuscitation: is one better? A randomized clinical study. *Surgery* 1979;85:129-39.
34 Woittiez AJ. Restoration of colloid osmotic pressure in post operative intensive care patients. A randomised placebo controlled trial with albu-

SYSTEMATIC REVIEW (OF THERAPY) WORKSHEET: 1 of 2

Clinical question:

Are the results of this systematic review (systematic review) of therapy valid?

Did the review address a clearly focused question? How likely is it that the search strategy would have missed eligible trials?

Are the inclusion criteria clearly stated?

Are the inclusion criteria relating to population, intervention and comparison groups and outcome appropriate?

How likely is it that the conclusions are valid (i.e. Are the included studies good quality randomised controlled trials)?

If a meta-analysis was performed, were the included studies sufficiently homogeneous to make it appropriate to pool data?

Are the valid results of this systematic review important?

Translating odds ratios to NNTs. The numbers in the body of the table are the NNTs for the corresponding odds ratios at that particular patient's expected event rate (PEER).

		Odds ratios (OR)								
		0.9	0.85	0.8	0.75	0.7	0.65	0.6	0.55	0.5
Patient's expected event rate (PEER)	.05	209[1]	139	104	83	69	59	52	46	41[2]
	.10	110	73	54	43	36	31	27	24	21
	.20	61	40	30	24	20	17	14	13	11
	.30	46	30	22	18	14	12	10	9	8
	.40	40	26	19	15	12	10	9	8	7
	.50[3]	38	25	18	14	11	9	8	7	6
	.70	44	28	20	16	13	10	9	7	6
	.90	101[4]	64	46	34	27	22	18	15	12[5]

[1]The relative risk reduction (RRR) here is 10%.

[2]The RRR here is 49%.

[3]For any OR, NNT is lowest when PEER = .50.

[4]The RRR here is 1%.

[5]The RRR here is 9%.

		Odds ratios (OR)				
		1.1	1.2	1.3	1.4	1.5
Patient's expected event rate (PEER)	.05	212	106	71	54	43
	.10	112	57	38	29	23
	.20	64	33	22	17	14
	.30	49	25	17	13	11
	.40	43	23	16	12	10
	.50[6]	42	22	15	12	10
	.70	51	27	19	15	135
	.90	121	66	47	38	32

The numbers in the body of the table are the NNTs for the corresponding odds ratios at that particular patient's expected event rate (PEER). This table applies both when a good outcome is increased by therapy and when a side-effect is caused by therapy.

Can you apply this valid, important evidence from a systematic review in caring for your patient?

Do these results apply to your patient?

Are my patients so different from those in the review that there are likely to be important differences in treatment effect?

Is the intervention in the studies in the review sufficiently similar to the treatment that I am considering?

Are the outcome measures documented an adequate reflection of the outcomes of importance to my patients?

How great would the potential benefit of therapy actually be for your individual patient?

Method I: In the table on p 1, find the intersection of the closest odds ratio from the overview and the CER that is closest to your patient's expected event rate if they received the control treatment (PEER):

Method II: To calculate the NNT for any OR and PEER:

$$\text{NNT} = \frac{1 - \{\text{PEER} \times (1 - \text{OR})\}}{(1 - \text{PEER}) \times \text{PEER} \times (1 - \text{OR})}$$

Are your patient's values and preferences satisfied by the regimen and its consequences?

Does your patient and you have a clear assessment of their values and preferences?

Are they met by this regimen and its consequences?

Should you believe apparent qualitative differences in the efficacy of therapy in some subgroups of patients? Only if you can say 'yes' to all of the following:

Do they really make biologic and clinical sense?

Is the qualitative difference both clinically (beneficial for some but useless or harmful for others) and statistically significant?

Was this difference hypothesised before the study began (rather than the product of dredging the data), and has it been confirmed in other, independent studies?

Was this one of just a few subgroup analyses carried out in this study?

Additional notes

Clinical question:	In children with meningococcal septicaemia (who are critically ill), does albumin improve mortality compared to crystalloids?

Are the results of this systematic review (systematic review) of therapy valid?

Did the review address a clearly focused question?	**Yes.**
How likely is it that the search strategy would have missed eligible trials?	**Unlikely.**
Are the inclusion criteria clearly stated?	**Yes.**
Are the inclusion criteria relating to population, intervention and comparison groups and outcome appropriate?	**Yes, and clinical subgroups of hypoalbumin, hypovolaemia, and burns are pre-specified.**
How likely is it that the conclusions are valid (i.e. Are the included studies good quality randomised controlled trials)?	**Conclusions for no benefit are valid. Conclusions regarding increased mortality is not significant if only high quality trials included.**
If a meta-analysis was performed, were the included studies sufficiently homogeneous to make it appropriate to pool the data?	**Yes. No significant heterogeneity found.**

Are the valid results of this systematic review important?

Translating odds ratios to NNTs. The numbers in the body of the table are the NNTs for the corresponding odds ratios at that particular patient's expected event rate (PEER).

		Odds ratios (OR)								
		0.9	0.85	0.8	0.75	0.7	0.65	0.6	0.55	0.5
Patient's expected event rate (PEER)	.05	209[1]	139	104	83	69	59	52	46	41[2]
	.10	110	73	54	43	36	31	27	24	21
	.20	61	40	30	24	20	17	14	13	11
	.30	46	30	22	18	14	12	10	9	8
	.40	40	26	19	15	12	10	9	8	7
	.50[3]	38	25	18	14	11	9	8	7	6
	.70	44	28	20	16	13	10	9	7	6
	.90	101[4]	64	46	34	27	22	18	15	12[5]

[1]The relative risk reduction (RRR) here is 10%.

[2]The RRR here is 49%.

[3]For any OR, NNT is lowest when PEER = .50.

[4]The RRR here is 1%.

[5]The RRR here is 9%.

		Odds ratios (OR)				
		1.1	1.2	1.3	1.4	1.5
Patient's expected event rate (PEER)	.05	212	106	71	54	43
	.10	112	57	38	29	23
	.20	64	33	22	17	14
	.30	49	25	17	13	11
	.40	43	23	16	12	10
	.50[6]	42	22	15	12	10
	.70	51	27	19	15	135
	.90	121	66	47	38	32

The numbers in the body of the table are the NNTs for the corresponding odds ratios at that particular patient's expected event rate (PEER). This table applies both when a good outcome is increased by therapy and when a side-effect is caused by therapy.

Results: For hypovolaemia, pooled odds for mortality ratio is 1.46 for all studies and studies with adequate concealment OR = 1.39 with 95% confidence interval of 0.8 to 2.4. CI includes 1 so is not statistically significant. There could be a 20% reduction in mortality in patients given albumin or as much as a 240% increase.

There is no evidence from the systematic review that albumin offers any advantage over crystalloid in critically ill hypovolaemic patients.

Can you apply this valid, important evidence from a systematic review in caring for your patient?

Do these results apply to your patient?

Are my patients so different from those in the review that there are likely to be important differences in treatment effect?	**Possibly. No studies specifically looked at meningococcal sepsis. Need strong justification that my patients are so biologically different in view of the consistent lack of benefit in all clinical groups.**
Is the intervention in the studies in the review sufficiently similar to the treatment I am considering?	**Yes.**
Are the outcome measures documented an adequate reflection of the outcomes of importance to my patients?	**Yes.**

How great would the potential benefit of therapy actually be for your individual patient?

(Note: study gives relative risk not odds ratio).	**Looking at So's study (neonates) for CER = 16%** **Therefore risk in albumin group = 0.16 × 1.39** **= 0.22.** **Risk difference = 0.06** **NNH = 16**
Method I: In the table on p 1, find the intersection of the closest odds ratio from the overview and the CER that is closest to your patient's expected event rate if they received the control treatment (PEER):	**NNH = 14–23**

Method II: To calculate the NNT for any OR and PEER:

$$\text{NNT} = \frac{1 - \{\text{PEER} \times (1 - \text{OR})\}}{(1 - \text{PEER}) \times \text{PEER} \times (1 - \text{OR})}$$

Are your patient's values and preferences satisfied by the regimen and its consequences?

Does your patient and you have a clear assessment of their values and preferences?	**Yes, improved survival.**
Are they met by this regimen and its consequences?	**Don't know. Effects for children with meningococcal sepsis uncertain.**

Should you believe apparent qualitative differences in the efficacy of therapy in some subgroups of patients? Only if you can say 'yes' to all of the following:

Do they really make biologic and clinical sense?	**No differences, but subgroups make sense.**
Is the qualitative difference both clinically (beneficial for some but useless or harmful for others) and statistically significant?	**No difference.** **Paediatricians believe children with meningococcal disease have different pathophysiology, so results do not apply.**

Was this difference hypothesised before the study began (rather than the product of dredging the data), and has it been confirmed in other, independent studies?	**Yes.**
Was this one of just a few subgroup analyses carried out in this study?	**Yes.**

Additional notes

Full details of studies are available from the Cochrane library with summaries of all results. Are children with meningococcal sepsis so different that results don't apply? PICU* experts would argue that they are. However, studies in a wide range of patient groups provide no evidence that albumin is more beneficial than crystalloids, and the evidence suggests that it may increase mortality. We need a randomised controlled trial of albumin versus crystalloids in critically ill children with meningococcal sepsis to provide the evidence.

*See Nadel *et al.* (1998) Albumin: saint or sinner? *Arch Dis Child* **79**(5): 384–5.

CRITICALLY ILL PATIENTS – ALBUMIN OF NO PROVEN BENEFIT

Appraised by O Duperrex and R Gilbert: 5 March 1999
Expiry date: March 2000.

Clinical Bottom Line

There is no evidence from research regarding the use of albumin in children with meningococcal sepsis. RCTs of albumin vs. crystalloids in children with meningococcal sepsis are needed. None of the trials in a wide range of patients show any benefit of albumin over crystalloids, and evidence suggests that albumin may increase mortality.

Citation

Cochrane Injuries Group Albumin Reviewers (Alderson P, Bunn F, Lefebvre C, Li Wan Po A, Li L, Roberts I and Schierhout G (1998) Human albumin administration in critically ill patients: systematic review of randomised controlled trials. *BMJ* **317:** 235–40.

For additional information see:

The Albumin Reviewers (1998) Human albumin administration in critically ill patients (Cochrane Review). In: *The Cochrane Library*, **Issue 3.** Oxford: Updated Software.

Clinical Question

In children with meningococcal sepsis (who are critically ill), does albumin improve mortality compared to crystalloids?

Search Terms

'meningococcal sepsis' and 'child' and 'albumin' and 'randomised-controlled-trial'.

The Study

Systematic review of 30 RCTs, including 1419 randomised patients. Only three studies included children.

The Evidence

Pooled relative risk of albumin vs. control for hypovolaemia in studies with adequate concealment was 1.39 (95% CI 0.8–2.4).

If baseline risk (PEER) is 16% (from the only study on hypovolaemia in premature babies), then NNH is 16. Or we could avoid 1 death for every 16 patients treated with crystalloids instead of albumin.

Comments

1 Five studies involved children who were premature (4) or burned (1). None specifically looked at patients with meningococcal sepsis.
2 There was no heterogeneity between studies.
3 There is no evidence that albumin is more beneficial than crystalliods for any of the indications (hypovolaemia, hypoalbuminaemia or burns). Use of albumin may increase mortality, is more costly and can transmit infection (it is a blood product).

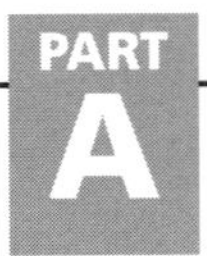

Critical appraisal of a clinical article about harm

EBCH SESSION

5

Harm and searching for evidence on the Web

Scenario: Vitamin A supplements and pregnancy

You are a midwife. During your antenatal classes, a woman asks whether it is safe to take vitamin A supplements as she has heard that there may be a risk of birth defects from supplements containing vitamin A. She wants your advice on what to do regarding vitamin supplementation.

You tell her you will investigate and you form the question, do pregnant women receiving vitamin A supplements have a higher risk of children having birth defects? You go to the library and search MEDLINE and find the enclosed article (*NEJM* 1995; 333: 1369–73).

What is your advice to her regarding vitamin A supplements?

Search strategy for Vitamin A and pregnancy

Type in: Vitamin A. You will see 'exp retinoids'
Type in:
1 exp retinoids
2 exp abnormalities
3 #1 and #2
4 exp pregnancy
5 #3 and #4
6 limit #5 to human
7 vitamin a.tw.
8 #6 and #7

Read this article and decide:
1 Are the results of this harm study valid?
2 Are the results of this harm study important?
3 Should these valid, important results of this study about a potentially harmful treatment change the treatment of your patient?

If you want to read some strategies for answering these sorts of questions, you could have a look at pp 105–10, 147–49 and 179–81 in *Evidence-based Medicine*.

PART B

Searching for evidence on the Web

We'll show you how to access the Web and introduce you to some interesting websites where there are databanks of useful information such as SpPins, SnNouts, likelihood ratios, and NNTs.

To help us organise your presentations for Sessions 6 and 7, please complete and hand in the form on the next page.

CASE PRESENTATION

My tentative clinical question:

My name:____

Contact address:____________________________________

Contact phone number:______________________________

Bleep:_______________

E-mail:____

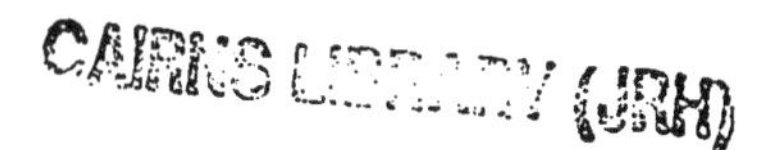

The New England Journal of Medicine

Volume 333 | NOVEMBER 23, 1995 | Number 21

TERATOGENICITY OF HIGH VITAMIN A INTAKE

KENNETH J. ROTHMAN, DR.P.H., LYNN L. MOORE, D.SC., MARTHA R. SINGER, M.P.H., R.D., TUYEN-SA D.T. NGUYEN, M.P.H., SALVATORE MANNINO, M.D., M.P.H., AND AUBREY MILUNSKY, M.B., B.CH., D.SC.

Abstract *Background.* Studies in animals indicate that natural forms of vitamin A are teratogenic. Synthetic retinoids chemically similar to vitamin A cause birth defects in humans; as in animals, the defects appear to affect tissues derived from the cranial neural crest.

Methods. Between October 1984 and June 1987, we identified 22,748 pregnant women when they underwent screening either by measurement of maternal serum alpha-fetoprotein or by amniocentesis. Nurse interviewers obtained information on the women's diet, medications, and illnesses during the first trimester of pregnancy, as well as information on their family and medical history and exposure to environmental agents. We obtained information on the outcomes of pregnancy from the obstetricians who delivered the babies or from the women themselves. Of the 22,748 women, 339 had babies with birth defects; 121 of these babies had defects occurring in sites that originated in the cranial neural crest.

Results. For defects associated with cranial-neural-crest tissue, the ratio of the prevalence among the babies born to women who consumed more than 15,000 IU of preformed vitamin A per day from food and supplements to the prevalence among the babies whose mothers consumed 5000 IU or less per day was 3.5 (95 percent confidence interval, 1.7 to 7.3). For vitamin A from supplements alone, the ratio of the prevalence among the babies born to women who consumed more than 10,000 IU per day to that among the babies whose mothers consumed 5000 IU or less per day was 4.8 (95 percent confidence interval, 2.2 to 10.5). Using a smoothed regression curve, we found an apparent threshold near 10,000 IU per day of supplemental vitamin A. The increased frequency of defects was concentrated among the babies born to women who had consumed high levels of vitamin A before the seventh week of gestation.

Conclusions. High dietary intake of preformed vitamin A appears to be teratogenic. Among the babies born to women who took more than 10,000 IU of preformed vitamin A per day in the form of supplements, we estimate that about 1 infant in 57 had a malformation attributable to the supplement. (N Engl J Med 1995;333:1369-73.)

VITAMIN A is essential for embryogenesis, growth, and epithelial differentiation. By the term "vitamin A," we refer to retinoid compounds that have the biologic activity of retinol. Preformed vitamin A in the diet comes from animal sources, such as dairy products and liver, and from fortified foods and vitamin supplements. Beta carotene and other carotenoids are plant-synthesized precursors of vitamin A that are partially converted to retinol during or after absorption.[1] Currently, the Recommended Dietary Allowance for women is 800 retinol equivalents, which corresponds to about 2700 IU of vitamin A per day.[2] In the United States, about 25 percent of adults ingest supplements containing vitamin A and about 5 percent take supplements of vitamin A alone.[3]

Experiments in animals have shown that retinoids (but not carotenoids) can be teratogenic.[1,4-6] In humans, isotretinoin, a synthetic retinoid used in the treatment of severe acne, causes congenital fetal anomalies.[7,8] Lammer et al. estimated that, with fetal exposure to isotretinoin, the risk of a malformation was 25 times greater than normal.[8] As in the studies in animals, a specific group of malformations ("retinoic acid embryopathy"), including those of craniofacial, cardiac, thymic, and central nervous system structures, appears to be involved.

Thus, the available evidence is consistent with the existence of a common teratogenic mechanism by which natural and synthetic retinoids affect the development of cephalic neural-crest cells and their derivatives and perhaps interfere with the closure of the neural tube.[8-14] Recent evidence indicates that the teratogenic effect of retinoids may derive from an effect on the expression of the homeobox gene *Hoxb-1* that regulates axial patterning in the embryo.[15,16]

Data on the teratogenicity of vitamin A in humans

From the Section of Preventive Medicine and Epidemiology, Evans Department of Medicine (K.J.R., L.L.M., M.R.S., T.-S.D.T.N.), and the Center for Human Genetics (A.M.), Boston University School of Medicine, Boston; and the Chair of Hygiene, Institute of Human Pathology and Social Medicine, University G. D'Annunzio, Chieti, Italy (S.M.). Address reprint requests to Dr. Rothman at Boston University School of Medicine, B-612, 88 E. Newton St., Boston, MA 02118.

Supported by a Public Health Service grant (NS 19561) from the National Institute of Neurological Disorders and Stroke and by a contract with F. Hoffmann-LaRoche, Ltd.

are scant.[17-21] Here we report on the relation between birth defects and the intake of vitamin A from food and supplements in a prospectively studied population of more than 22,000 pregnant women.

METHODS

The study cohort was originally recruited to evaluate risk factors for neural-tube defects.[22] Between October 1984 and June 1987, women from the practices of more than 100 participating obstetricians were identified when they either had a maternal serum alpha-fetoprotein measurement or underwent amniocentesis. The study protocol was reviewed and approved by the Boston University Medical Center's Institutional Review Board for Human Research.

Nearly all the women were enrolled between week 15 and week 20 of pregnancy. Nurse interviewers contacted the women by telephone to obtain information on diet, medications, and illnesses during the first trimester of pregnancy, as well as general information on their family and medical history and exposure to environmental and occupational agents. The interviewers called 24,559 women, of whom 23,491 gave their consent to participate. Of those interviewed, 29 women were excluded because their interviews were incomplete, 686 because they could not be located for follow-up, and 21 because information on the outcome of pregnancy was missing. These exclusions left 22,755 women with completed interviews and follow-up information.

Retinol Intake

The interviewers asked each woman detailed questions about her diet and her use of vitamin supplements. Women were asked, "In the three months prior to pregnancy, did you take a multivitamin?" Women who said yes were asked for the brand name of the vitamin and how many times it was taken each week. Each woman was then asked specifically whether she took supplements of vitamin A, vitamin C, vitamin E, nutritional yeast, folic acid, selenium, zinc, iron, or any other nutrient during the three months before she became pregnant. Then each woman was asked for similar information about the use of multivitamins and supplements during the first three months of her pregnancy, including the brand used, the week of pregnancy during which she began to take the vitamin, the frequency of use, and any changes in intake during this period. Information on the dosage of vitamin A was obtained from information on file about each multivitamin brand, or from the subject in the case of supplements of vitamin A alone. The timing of use during pregnancy was determined according to the reported date of the last menstrual period.

Some data on the multivitamin brand, the week vitamin use began, the frequency of intake, or the dosage of single-vitamin supplements were missing for 201 women. For these women, we substituted median values for the missing values. For example, if the week of first vitamin use was missing and the brand was a prenatal formulation, we used the median starting week for all users of prenatal vitamins. We also analyzed the data after excluding women for whom we had made such substitutions.

We estimated retinol intake during each of the 12 weeks since the last menstrual period for all the subjects for whom we had information on vitamin supplements, diet, and the outcome of pregnancy. For most analyses we classified retinol intake from food and supplements according to the mean amounts ingested during the four weeks of highest consumption during the first trimester.

The women were also asked about their consumption of 50 different foods, with this question: "How often, per day, per week, or per month, did you eat one serving of the following foods during the first eight weeks of your pregnancy?" Servings were defined by the interviewers for each food item (for example, one slice of cheese or half a grapefruit).

Our food-related analysis included only foods that are sources of retinol: milk, cheese, margarine, butter, eggs, mashed potatoes (which often contain butter and milk), chicken, chicken liver, beef, beef liver, processed meats, pizza, fish, and cold breakfast cereals. Since the women were asked to name up to three brands of breakfast cereal that they ate most often, we calculated an average retinol content for cereal based on the reported brands. We used the daily intake of retinol from each of the above foods to estimate the total daily intake of retinol from the diet.

For 106 women, information on some, but fewer than half, of the retinol-containing foods was missing. For these foods, we assigned values for retinol intake, using the median daily intake for all women in the study. We excluded from our analyses 6 women for whom information for half or more of the retinol-containing foods was missing and 1 woman for whom we lacked information on vitamin supplements; these additional exclusions left 22,748 women for whom we had completed interviews and usable data on retinol intake from both foods and vitamin supplements.

Outcome of Pregnancy

Information on the outcome of pregnancy was obtained from a questionnaire mailed to the obstetrician around the expected time of delivery. If the physician did not respond, the same questionnaire was mailed to the mother. Information requested on the follow-up form included the presence of any birth defects as well as other information about complications and outcome of pregnancy. Physicians supplied the information for 76.5 percent of the pregnancies; the mothers supplied the information for the remainder.

Two coders reviewed the outcome forms, independently classifying reported birth defects according to the codes of the Centers for Disease Control and Prevention manual for birth-defect classification.[23] In cases of disagreement, a third coder examined the data and made a final decision about outcome codes. During the coding, all coders were unaware of the dietary information provided by the mothers. After coding, we classified each defect into one of the following categories: craniofacial defects (e.g., oral clefts and anomalies of the ears, eyes, and nose); central nervous system defects (e.g., reduction deformities of the brain, microcephaly, and hydrocephaly in the absence of spina bifida); anomalies of the thymus; heart defects; neural-tube defects (spina bifida, anencephaly, and encephalocele); musculoskeletal defects (limb-reduction deformities, clubfoot, syndactyly, polydactyly, and other bony defects of shoulder, forearm, wrist, and hand); urogenital defects (e.g., renal agenesis, congenital hydronephrosis, other defects of the kidneys, anomalies of the external genitalia, and hypospadias); defects of the digestive tract (e.g., tracheoesophageal fistula, congenital hypertrophic pyloric stenosis, and atresia or stenosis of intestines); and other defects (e.g., agenesis or hypoplasia of the lungs, single umbilical artery, anomalies of the spleen, and cystic hygroma).

In classifying babies with more than one birth defect, we counted each baby only once, using the following hierarchy, in descending order of priority: craniofacial, central nervous system, or thymic defects; heart defects; neural-tube defects; musculoskeletal defects; urogenital defects; defects of the digestive tract; and other defects. We did not code chromosomal defects or malformations stemming from genetic causes, such as Tay–Sachs disease or cystic fibrosis, nor did we include cerebral palsy, malabsorption syndrome, a limb defect reportedly caused by an amniotic band, or conditions that were listed as birth defects on the forms but were clearly not malformations.

Craniofacial, central nervous system, thymic, and heart defects arise, at least in part, from cranial-neural-crest cells. We grouped these defects as cranial-neural-crest outcomes. We considered neural-tube defects separately; we also considered musculoskeletal and urogenital defects separately, because in some reports they have been found to be related to retinoids.[7] We grouped gastrointestinal and all other defects listed above into the fourth outcome category, "other defects."

Statistical Analysis

We analyzed the data first by obtaining contingency tables for the main study variables, from which we calculated the prevalence of birth defects according to the mothers' retinol-intake category, along with prevalence ratios and approximate 95 percent confidence intervals.[24] We then stratified the contingency tables according to each of several possible confounding variables, which included the age, education, and race of the mother and the maternal history or family history of birth defects. We also fitted a multiple logistic-regression model to the data that controlled for the above variables as well as folate intake, alcohol consumption, genital herpes infection, treated maternal diabetes, fever (temperature, ≥38.3°C [101°F]) during the first trimester of pregnancy, and the use of antiseizure medication, retinoids, or exogenous hormones.[24]

High vitamin A intake from supplements can result from taking a multivitamin with a high vitamin A content (some contained as much as 25,000 IU), from taking more than one multivitamin pill per day with a smaller dose of vitamin A, from taking vitamin A supplements, or from some combination of these. For analyses of supplement use, we used an intake of more than 10,000 IU of retinol from supplements as the highest dose category, because many multivitamin supplements contained as much as 10,000 IU in a single pill, and only a few contained more than 10,000 IU. To obtain a clearer picture of the shape of the dose–prevalence relation, we used quadratic splines to smooth the dose–prevalence curve.[25]

Results

Among the 22,748 women in this analysis, 339 had babies with birth defects that met our study criteria. Of these, 121 were of cranial-neural-crest origin. The distribution of these birth defects according to major category is shown in Table 1.

Most women who took supplements containing vitamin A took multivitamins that contained retinol. There were 131 women, however, who took supplements of pure retinol, of whom 100 took multivitamin supplements as well. The distribution of total daily retinol consumption (from food and both types of supplements) for the entire cohort is shown in Table 2, along with the frequency of cranial-neural-crest and other birth defects in each of four categories of retinol consumption.

As Table 2 shows, the proportion of babies born with birth defects appeared to be relatively constant for the first three categories of total retinol intake, but the women who consumed more than 15,000 IU of retinol per day had a higher proportion of babies with birth defects. For defects associated with cranial-neural-crest tissue, the ratio of the prevalence among the babies born to women who consumed more than 15,000 IU per day to the prevalence among the babies born to women who consumed 5000 IU or less per day was 3.5 (95 percent confidence interval, 1.7 to 7.3). There was a less striking trend for musculoskeletal and urogenital defects, and no discernible trend for neural-tube defects or other birth defects. For all birth defects combined, the prevalence ratio was 2.2 (95 percent confidence interval, 1.3 to 3.8).

When we cross-classified retinol intake from food and intake from supplements, we found that the distribution of intake from food was nearly uncorrelated with the intake from supplements ($r = 0.005$). We therefore proceeded to examine retinol intake from supplements and from food separately (Table 3). Few women consumed large amounts of retinol from food alone. Among those who did, there was some indication of an increase in the prevalence of birth defects for those who consumed the highest amounts of retinol, but the small numbers make the estimate imprecise. The prevalence ratio for all birth defects among babies born to women who consumed more than 10,000 IU per day from food alone, as compared with the babies whose mothers consumed 5000 IU or less per day, was 1.8 (95 percent confidence interval, 0.8 to 4.3). For defects related to the cranial neural crest, the prevalence ratio was 2.0, but this ratio is statistically unstable, since it is based on only two cases of birth defects in babies born to women in the high retinol-intake category.

The effect of retinol from supplements was more striking. For all birth defects, the prevalence ratio for the babies born to women who consumed more than 10,000 IU per day as compared with the babies born to women who consumed 5000 IU or less per day was 2.4 (95 percent confidence interval, 1.3 to 4.4). For defects associated with cranial-neural-crest tissue, the corresponding prevalence ratio was 4.8 (95 percent confidence interval, 2.2 to 10.5). There was a progressive increase in the prevalence of cranial-neural-crest defects and in total birth defects from the lowest to the highest intake categories. We used the midpoints of the categories and, for the highest category, the mean intake (21,675 IU) to obtain the least-squares linear regression for the trend in cranial-neural-crest defects. From the regression we estimated that the prevalence of cranial-neural-crest defects increased by 0.00065 for each increase of 1000 IU in the daily intake of vitamin A from supplements (95 percent confidence interval, 0.00032 to 0.00097). The prevalence of cranial-neural-crest defects in the highest intake category was greater

Table 1. Birth Defects According to Category.

Type of Defect	No.
Cranial neural crest	
Craniofacial, central nervous system (except neural tube), and thymic	69
Heart	52
Total	121
Neural tube	48
Musculoskeletal and urogenital	
Musculoskeletal	58
Urogenital	42
Total	100
Other	
Gastrointestinal	24
Nongastrointestinal	46
Total	70
Total	339

Table 2. Pregnancies Resulting in Birth Defects, According to Daily Intake of Retinol from Food and Supplements Combined.

Daily Retinol Intake	Total Pregnancies	Cranial-Neural-Crest Defects	Neural-Tube Defects	Musculoskeletal or Urogenital Defects	Other Defects	Total Defects
IU	*no.*			*number (percent)*		
0–5000	6,410	33 (0.51)	13 (0.20)	24 (0.37)	16 (0.25)	86 (1.3)
5001–10,000	12,688	59 (0.47)	29 (0.23)	62 (0.49)	46 (0.36)	196 (1.5)
10,001–15,000	3,150	20 (0.63)	5 (0.16)	10 (0.32)	7 (0.22)	42 (1.3)
≥15,001	500	9 (1.80)	1 (0.20)	4 (0.80)	1 (0.20)	15 (3.0)

Table 3. Pregnancies Resulting in Birth Defects, According to Category of Daily Retinol Intake and Source of Retinol.

Daily Retinol Intake	Total Pregnancies	Cranial-Neural-Crest Defects	Neural-Tube Defects	Musculoskeletal or Urogenital Defects	Other Defects	Total Defects
IU	*no.*	*number (percent)*				
From food						
0–5000	21,755	114 (0.52)	44 (0.20)	95 (0.44)	67 (0.31)	320 (1.5)
5001–10,000	805	5 (0.62)	3 (0.37)	3 (0.37)	3 (0.37)	14 (1.7)
≥10,001	188	2 (1.06)	1 (0.53)	2 (1.06)	0	5 (2.7)
From supplements						
0–5000	11,083	51 (0.46)	21 (0.19)	44 (0.40)	32 (0.29)	148 (1.3)
5001–8000	10,585	54 (0.51)	26 (0.25)	52 (0.49)	36 (0.34)	168 (1.6)
8001–10,000	763	9 (1.18)	1 (0.13)	2 (0.26)	1 (0.13)	13 (1.7)
≥10,001	317	7 (2.21)	0	2 (0.63)	1 (0.32)	10 (3.2)

than the prevalence in the lowest intake category by 1.7 percent of births, or 1 baby in 57.

We then evaluated the effects of a high intake of vitamin A from food and supplements after stratifying the data according to potential confounding factors. We found little confounding by any single factor. We also constructed several multiple logistic-regression models incorporating vitamin A intake from food and supplements, with additional terms for the age, education, and race of the mother, the family history of birth defects, use of folate supplements during early pregnancy, treated maternal diabetes, alcohol consumption, genital herpes infection, fever (temperature, ≥38.3°C during the first trimester), and use of antiseizure medication, retinoids, or exogenous hormones. The estimates of the effects of vitamin A from both food and supplements were similar to the corresponding estimates from Table 3, even when both factors were in the same model. Thus, there was little aggregate confounding from the factors mentioned.

To improve our estimate of the shape of the dose–response curve relating the intake of supplements to the occurrence of cranial-neural-crest defects, we fitted an unrestricted quadratic-spline logistic model, using the same four intake categories and the same terms for all the potential confounding variables cited above. The smoothed exposure–effect curve, shown in Figure 1, indicates an apparent threshold near 10,000 IU of vitamin A per day from supplements. The figure also shows the curve for total retinol, which rises more slowly.

To evaluate how the timing of vitamin A intake affected the risk of cranial-neural-crest defects, we examined the prevalence of defects among the babies born to women whose average daily vitamin A intake exceeded 10,000 IU during three mutually exclusive time periods before conception and during early gestation (Table 4). These findings indicate a high prevalence of birth defects related to the cranial neural crest in association with high levels of exposure before or during organ formation, but not after.

The seven babies with cranial-neural-crest defects who were born to mothers in the highest category of supplemental retinol intake (Table 3) had the following defects: cleft lip, ventricular septal defect, transposition of the great vessels, hydrocephaly (two babies), multiple heart defects, and craniosynostosis. All seven mothers took high doses of vitamin A from supplements in the two weeks before conception or during the first month of pregnancy.

Some pregnancies included in our denominator ended in early fetal death. If these early terminations of pregnancy were unequally distributed among the categories of retinol intake, it could have biased our findings. To evaluate this possibility, we reanalyzed the data after excluding these pregnancies. The results were nearly identical to the results without these exclusions. We also reanalyzed the data with all early terminations considered as adverse events and found a similar pattern of effects. When we omitted women for whom data substitutions were used to determine vitamin A intake, the results changed very little.

Discussion

Our findings indicate that vitamin A is potentially teratogenic, but these findings relate solely to preformed vitamin A and not to beta carotene, a vitamin A precursor. We did not study beta carotene specifically, but studies in animals indicate that a high intake of beta carotene is neither toxic nor teratogenic.[1,3-6]

A relation between high vitamin A consumption during early pregnancy and the occurrence of birth defects is consistent with the results of studies of retinol in animals[4,5] and of the effects of isotretinoin in humans[7,8] and with two earlier case–control studies.[20,21] The strong

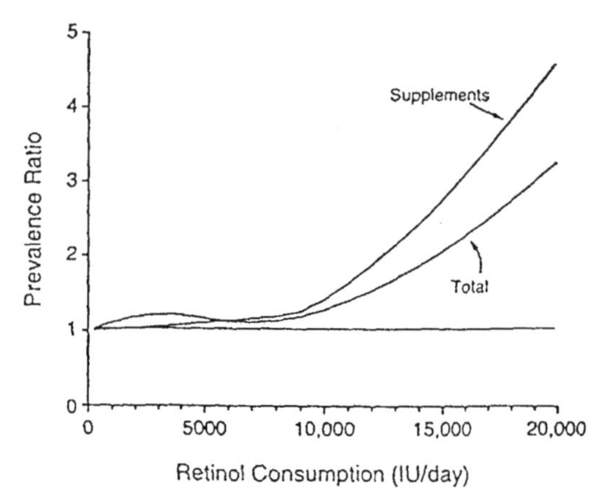

Figure 1. Estimated Prevalence Ratio for Birth Defects Related to the Cranial Neural Crest, According to Retinol Intake during the First Trimester of Pregnancy.

The smoothed curves were fitted with unrestricted quadratic splines. The prevalence ratio is the ratio of the prevalence of defects among the babies born to women who consumed a given amount of vitamin A (from food and supplements [total] or from supplements alone) to the prevalence among the babies of women with a hypothetical intake of zero.

Table 4. Cranial-Neural-Crest Defects among Babies Born to Women Taking More Than 10,000 IU of Vitamin A per Day from Supplements, According to the Timing of High Intake.*

Variable	High Intake Only during 2 Weeks before Conception	High Intake Only before Week 7 of Pregnancy	High Intake Only after Week 6 of Pregnancy
Cranial-neural-crest defects (no.)	2	3	0
Pregnancies (no.)	42	80	70
Prevalence (%)	4.8	3.8	0

*The three periods are mutually exclusive.

effect of high levels of retinol intake from supplements in our study is not easily ascribed to confounding or information bias. The stronger relation seen for vitamin A taken before or during organ formation than for vitamin A taken later is also consistent with a causal effect, but not with any plausible reporting bias. The apparently weaker relation between birth defects and retinol from food, as compared with supplements, may reflect greater error in measuring vitamin A levels in food or lower bioavailability of retinol consumed during meals.

These data appear to indicate a teratogenic effect of vitamin A at levels not far above those currently recommended. In our study population, about 1.4 percent of women averaged more than 10,000 IU of vitamin A per day from supplements. Since these data were collected, some manufacturers have decreased the retinol content of multivitamins, often substituting beta carotene. These changes may have lessened the teratogenic effects of vitamin A in the population as a whole. Among women who take more than 10,000 IU of preformed vitamin A per day from supplements, we estimate that 1 of every 57 babies is born with a birth defect attributable to the high vitamin A intake of the mother.

We are indebted to Dr. Peter Glasner for his advice, to the Boston Collaborative Drug Surveillance Program for its key role in the research effort, and to Dr. Quirino Orlandi for help with the birth-defect coding.

References

1. Bendich A, Langseth L. Safety of vitamin A. Am J Clin Nutr 1989;49:358-71.
2. National Research Council. Recommended dietary allowances. 10th ed. Washington, D.C.: National Academy Press, 1989:84.
3. Hathcock JN, Hattan DG, Jenkins MY, McDonald JT, Sundaresan PR, Wilkening VL. Evaluation of vitamin A toxicity. Am J Clin Nutr 1990;52:183-202.
4. Cohlan SQ. Congenital anomalies in the rat produced by excessive intake of vitamin A during pregnancy. Pediatrics 1954;13:556-67.
5. Geelen JA. Hypervitaminosis A induced teratogenesis. Crit Rev Toxicol 1979;6:351-75.
6. Pinnock CB, Alderman CP. The potential for teratogenicity of vitamin A and its congeners. Med J Aust 1992;157:804-9.
7. Rosa FW. Teratogenicity of isotretinoin. Lancet 1983;2:513.
8. Lammer EJ, Chen DT, Hoar RM, et al. Retinoic acid embryopathy. N Engl J Med 1985;313:837-41.
9. Use of supplements containing high-dose vitamin A — New York State, 1983-1984. MMWR Morb Mortal Wkly Rep 1987;36:80-2.
10. Teratology Society position paper: recommendations for vitamin A use during pregnancy. Teratology 1987;35:269-75.
11. Kirby ML. Cardiac morphogenesis — recent research advances. Pediatr Res 1987;21:219-24.
12. Bockman DE, Kirby ML. Dependence of thymus development on derivatives of the neural crest. Science 1984;223:498-500.
13. Dencker L, Gustafson AL, Annerwall E, Busch C, Eriksson U. Retinoid-binding proteins in craniofacial development. J Craniofac Genet Dev Biol 1991;11:303-14.
14. Eckhoff CH, Nau H. Vitamin A supplementation increases levels of retinoic acid compounds in human plasma: possible implications for teratogenesis. Arch Toxicol 1990;64:502-3.
15. Marshall H, Studer M, Pöpperl H, et al. A conserved retinoic acid response element required for early expression of the homeobox gene *Hoxb-1*. Nature 1994;370:567-71.
16. Studer M, Pöpperl H, Marshall H, Kuriowa A, Krumlauf R. Role of a conserved retinoic acid response element in rhombomere restriction of *Hoxb-1*. Science 1994;265:1728-32.
17. Rosa FW, Wilk AL, Kelsey FO. Teratogen update: vitamin A congeners. Teratology 1986;33:355-64.
18. Evans K, Hickey-Dwyer MU. Cleft anterior segment with maternal hypervitaminosis A. Br J Ophthalmol 1991;75:691-2.
19. Kizer KW, Fan AM, Bankowska J, Jackson RJ, Lyman DO. Vitamin A — a pregnancy alert. West J Med 1990;152:78-81.
20. Werler MW, Lammer EJ, Rosenberg L, Mitchell AA. Maternal vitamin A supplementation in relation to selected birth defects. Teratology 1990;42:497-503.
21. Martínez-Frías ML, Salvador J. Epidemiological aspects of prenatal exposure to high doses of vitamin A in Spain. Eur J Epidemiol 1990;6:118-23.
22. Milunsky A, Jick H, Jick SS, et al. Multivitamin/folic acid supplementation in early pregnancy reduces the prevalence of neural tube defects. JAMA 1989;262:2847-52.
23. Centers for Disease Control. Birth defects branch six digit code. Document No. 0025M. Atlanta: Centers for Disease Control, 1985.
24. Rothman KJ. Modern epidemiology. Boston: Little, Brown, 1986.
25. Greenland S. Dose-response and trend analysis in epidemiology: alternatives to categorical analysis. Epidemiology 1995;6:356-65.

HARM/AETIOLOGY WORKSHEET: 1 of 2

Clinical question:

Are the results of this harm study valid?

Were there clearly defined groups of patients, similar in all important ways other than exposure to the treatment or other cause?

Were treatment exposures and clinical outcomes measured the same ways in both groups, e.g. was the assessment of outcomes either objective (e.g. death) or blinded to exposure?

Was the follow-up of study patients complete and long enough?

Do the results satisfy some 'diagnostic tests for causation'?

- Is it clear that the exposure preceded the onset of the outcome?
- Is there a dose-response gradient?
- Is there positive evidence from a 'dechallenge-rechallenge' study?
- Is the association consistent from study to study?
- Does the association make biological sense?

Are the valid results from this harm study important?

		Adverse outcome		Totals
		Present (case)	**Absent (control)**	
Exposed to the treatment	Yes (Cohort)	a	b	a + b
	No (Cohort)	c	d	c + d
	Totals	a + c	b + d	a + b + c + d

In a randomised trial or cohort study: relative risk = RR = [a/(a + b)]/[c/(c + d)]

In a case-control study: odds ratio (or relative odds) = OR = ad/bc

In this study:

HARM/AETIOLOGY WORKSHEET: 2 of 2

Should these valid, potentially important results of a critical appraisal about a harmful treatment change the treatment of your patient?

Can the study results be extrapolated to your patient?

What are your patient's risks of the adverse outcome?
To calculate the NNH[1] for any odds ratio (OR) and your patient's expected event rate for this adverse event if they were **not** exposed to this treatment (PEER):

$$NNH = \frac{PEER\,(OR - 1) + 1}{PEER\,(OR - 1) \times (1 - PEER)}$$

What are your patient's preferences, concerns and expectations from this treatment?

What alternative treatments are available?

---

[1]The number of patients you need to treat to harm one of them.

Additional notes

COMPLETED HARM/AETIOLOGY WORKSHEET: 1 of 2

Clinical question: In pregnancy, does taking Vitamin A supplements increase the risk of birth defects?

Are the results of this harm study valid?	
Were there clearly defined groups of patients, similar in all important ways other than exposure to the treatment or other cause?	**Yes. Cohort of 22 748 pregnant women.**
Were treatment exposures and clinical outcomes measured the same ways in both groups, e.g. was the assessment of outcomes either objective (death) or blinded to exposure?	**Yes. All were interviewed regarding diet etc. early in pregnancy. Everyone was blind to outcome (birth defects) and birth defects were clearly defined.**
Was the follow-up of study patients complete and long enough?	**Yes. 96.8% follow-up.**
Do the results satisfy some 'diagnostic tests for causation'?	
• Is it clear that the exposure preceded the onset of the outcome?	**Yes. Vitamin A before conception and in the early weeks of pregnancy.**
• Is there a dose-response gradient?	**Yes. See Fig. 1.**
• Is there positive evidence from a 'dechallenge-rechallenge' study?	**No.**
• Is the association consistent from study to study?	**Yes. See last paragraph of p 1369. Results similar to those from animal studies and synthetic retinoids.**
• IDoes the association make biologic sense?	**Yes.**

COMPLETED HARM/AETIOLOGY WORKSHEET: 2 of 2

Are the valid results from this harm study important?

		Adverse outcome (CNC defects)		Totals
		Present (case)	**Absent (control)**	
Exposed to the treatment	Yes (>10 000 iu/day)	7 a	310 b	317 a + b
	No (<5000 iu/day)	51 c	11 032 d	11 083 c + d
	Totals	58 a + c	11 342 b + d	11 400 a + b + c + d

From Table 3 for vitamin A supplements.

Relative risk = [7/317]/[51/11083] = 0.022/0.0046 = 4.8

Should these valid, potentially important results of a critical appraisal about a harmful treatment change the treatment of your patient?

Can the study results be extrapolated to your patient?	**Yes.**
What are your patient's risks of the adverse outcome? To calculate the NNH[1] for any odds ratio (OR) and your patient's expected event rate for this adverse event if they were **not** exposed to this treatment (PEER): $$NNH = \frac{PEER\ (OR - 1) + 1}{PEER\ (OR - 1) \times (1 - PEER)}$$ Assume your PEER as same as in the study.	**Risk with suppl. >10 000 = 7/317 = 0.022** **Risk with suppl. <5000 = 51/11083 = 0.005** **ARI with suppl. >10 000 = 0.022–0.005 = 0.017** **NNH = 1/ARI = 1/0.017 = 59**
What are your patient's preferences, concerns and expectations from this treatment?	**Mother must balance potential benefits for her own health with risks of high doses to her baby's health.**
What alternative treatments are available?	**She can take low dose supplements (i.e. <5000 iu vitamin A/day)**

[1]The number of patients you need to treat to harm one of them.

Additional notes

If you look at cranial-neural crest defects (CNC) and vitamin A supplements, RR is 4.8 (i.e. nearly fivefold increase in the risk of CNC defects) in women taking supplements >10 000 iu vitamin A/day compared to <5000 iu vitamin A/day.

You can work out the 95% CI around the RR for vitamin A supplements and CNC defects. 95% CI are 2.2 to 10.5 which does not include 1 so is statistically significant and clinically important.

NEURAL TUBE DEFECTS – VITAMIN A IN PREGNANCY INCREASES THE RISK

Appraised by O Duperrex and R Gilbert: 5 March 1999
Expiry date: March 2000.

Clinical Bottom Line

Pregnant women taking supplements of vitamin A >10 000 iu/day increase their risk of having a child with cranial neural crest (CNC) defect by nearly 5 times (NNH = 57 with a baseline risk of 0.5%).

Citation

Rothman KJ, Moore LL, Singer MR et al. (1995) Teratogenicity of high vitamin A intake. *NEJM* **333**(21): 1369–73.

Clinical Question

Do pregnant women receiving vitamin A supplements have a higher risk of having children with birth defects?

Search Terms

'retinoids' and 'abnormalities' and 'pregnancy'

The Study

1 Cohort study of pregnant women being screened by AFP or amniocentesis (23 491 out of 24 559 gave consent to participate), outcomes known for 22 748 (96.8%).
2 Exposure assessed between week 15 and week 20 (since last menstruation) by telephone interview performed by nurse (blind to outcome) with detailed questions on diet, medications and illnesses during first trimester, allowing calculation of estimated daily vitamin A intake.
3 Outcome was obtained around expected time of delivery from obstetricians (76.5%) and mothers (23.5%) by questionnaire and then classified by blinded coders. Disagreements were submitted to a third coder.

The Evidence

Outcome	EER[1]	CER[2]	RR[3] (95%CI)	ARI	NNH (95%CI)
All birth defects	0.031	0.013	2.3 (2.36–2.45)	1.8%	55 (30–1250)
CNC defects	0.022	0.005	4.8 (2.2–10.5)	1.7%	59 (NNT 2044 to infinity; NNH 26 to infinity)

[1]Vitamin A >15 000 iu/day.
[2]Vitamin A ≤5 000 iu/day.
[3]Called 'prevalence ratio' in paper.

Comments

1 The risk is only associated with preformed vitamin A supplement not beta carotene.
2 There was a dose-response gradient.
3 There was no statistically significant association between cranial neural crest defects and high vitamin A intake from food only.

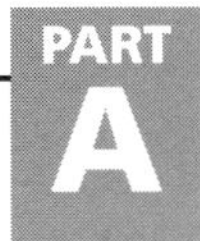

Presentations (comfortably 3 per hour)

1 In groups of 10 or less, participants will present their critical appraisals they have carried out on clinical topics of their choice.
2 Reports will state the three-part clinical question, summarise the search in one sentence, critically appraise the best article found, and discuss how the appraisal was integrated with clinical expertise and applied on that (or a similar, subsequent) patient.
3 A total of 15 minutes will be allotted for each presentation: 10 minutes for presentation and 5 minutes for group discussion.

EBCH SESSION 6

Presentations and searching the Cochrane Library

PART B

Searching the Cochrane Library

We will show you how to search the Cochrane Library (an electronic database of thousands of systematic reviews by the Cochrane Collaboration, abstracts of other systematic reviews from the world literature, citations for several hundred thousand randomised trials, and lots of information about the Cochrane Collaboration).

The Cochrane Library can be ordered from the BMJ Publishing Group (PO Box 295, London WC1H 9TE; Phone 0171-387-4499 and ask for 'Subscriptions'; Fax: 0171-383-6662; email: bmjsubs@dial.pipex.com).

EBCH SESSION 7

Presentations, feedback and celebration

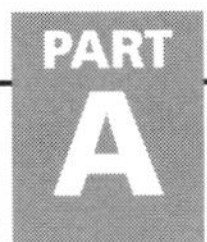

Part A Presentations

The other half of the participants will present their patients, questions, critically appraised topics, and clinical conclusions.

Part B Feedback and Celebration

The final portion of the session (and course!) can be spent evaluating the course. The first of the attached forms (**'Evaluation of 'practising *EBCH*''**) permits written feedback about this course, and a discussion will be held on the general issues within it.

The second form (**'Am I practising EBCH?'**) is a checklist that you may want to apply to your own performance in order to determine whether you are beginning to apply the self-directed, problem-based learning and EBCH skills in your own practice and in your clinical teaching.

Special attention will be given to discussing and deciding what to do with what has been learned, and how to continue to improve and use this set of clinical, EBM and self-directed learning skills.

EVALUATION OF 'PRACTISING EBM'

Please rate the items using the following scale from 1 to 5 where:

1 – awful 3 – adequate 5 – excellent

1 *How well were your objectives met in this course?*

a Learning how to ask answerable clinical questions related to pts you care for on the clinical service
1 2 3 4 5

b Learning how to search for the best evidence
1 2 3 4 5

c Learning how to critically appraise the medical literature
1 2 3 4 5

d Learning how to integrate this literature with your clinical expertise and to apply the results in your clinical practice
1 2 3 4 5

e Learning how to evaluate your performance
1 2 3 4 5

2 *Therapy Session*

a	Relevance of the session	1	2	3	4	5
b	Appropriateness of the article	1	2	3	4	5
c	Organisation of the session	1	2	3	4	5
d	Teaching during the session	1	2	3	4	5

3 *Diagnosis Session*

a	Relevance of the session	1	2	3	4	5
b	Appropriateness of the article	1	2	3	4	5
c	Organisation of the session	1	2	3	4	5
d	Teaching during the session	1	2	3	4	5

3 *Prognosis Session*

a	Relevance of the session	1	2	3	4	5
b	Appropriateness of the article	1	2	3	4	5
c	Organisation of the session	1	2	3	4	5
d	Teaching during the session	1	2	3	4	5

4 *Systematic Review Session*

a	Relevance of the session	1	2	3	4	5
b	Appropriateness of the article	1	2	3	4	5
c	Organisation of the session	1	2	3	4	5
d	Teaching during the session	1	2	3	4	5

5 *Harm Session*

a	Relevance of the session	1	2	3	4	5
b	Appropriateness of the article	1	2	3	4	5
c	Organisation of the session	1	2	3	4	5
d	Teaching during the session	1	2	3	4	5

6 *Final Presentation Sessions*

a	Relevance of the presentations	1	2	3	4	5
b	Quality of the presentations	1	2	3	4	5
c	Quality of the discussions	1	2	3	4	5
d	Organisation of the session	1	2	3	4	5

7 *How well do you think this course will help you prepare for your Membership Exams?*

1 2 3 4 5

8 *Overall rating of the course*

1 2 3 4 5

9 *What was the best thing about this course (that should be preserved and expanded in future courses)?*

10 *What was the worst thing about this course (that should be removed from future courses of this sort)?*

11 *Other comments and suggestions:*

Many thanks

AM I PRACTISING EBM?

A self-evaluation in asking answerable questions.

a Are you asking any questions at all?

b Are you:

- using the guides to asking 3-part questions?
- using educational prescriptions
- asking your colleagues: 'What's your evidence for that?'

c Is your success rate of asking answerable questions rising?

d How do your questions compare with those of respected colleagues?

A self-evaluation in finding the best external evidence.

a Are you searching at all?

b Do you know the best sources of current evidence for your clinical discipline?

c Have you achieved immediate access to searching hardware, software and the best evidence for your clinical discipline?

d Are you finding useful external evidence from a widening array of sources?

e Are you becoming more efficient in your searching?

f Are you using MeSH headings, thesaurus, limiters, and intelligent free text when searching MEDLINE?

g How do your searches compare with those of research librarians or other respected colleagues who have a passion for providing best current patient care?

A self-evaluation in critically appraising the evidence for its validity and potential usefulness.

a Are you critically appraising external evidence at all?

b Are the critical appraisal guides becoming easier to apply?

c Are you becoming more accurate and efficient in applying some of the critical appraisal measures (such as likelihood ratios, NNTs and the like)?

d Are you creating any CATs?

e Are you using the CATMaker?

f Have you shared any of the CATs you've made with your colleagues or other learners?

A self-evaluation in integrating the critical appraisal with your clinical expertise and applying the result in your clinical practice.

a Are you integrating your critical appraisals into your practice at all?

b Are you becoming more accurate and efficient in adjusting some of the critical appraisal measures to fit your individual patients (pre-test probabilities, NNT/f, etc.)?

c Can you explain (and resolve) disagreements about management decisions in terms of this integration?

d Have you conducted any clinical decision analyses?

e Have you carried out any audits of your diagnostic, therapeutic, or other EBM performance?

A self-evaluation in teaching EBCH.

a When did you last issue an educational prescription?

b Are you helping your trainees learn how to ask answerable (3-part) questions?

c Are you teaching and modelling searching skills (or making sure that your trainees learn them)?

d Are you teaching and modelling critical appraisal skills?

e Are you teaching and modelling the generation of CATs?

f Are you teaching and modelling the integration of best evidence with individual clinical expertise?

g Are you developing new ways of evaluating the effectiveness of your teaching?[1]

h Are you developing new EBCH educational materials?[2]

A self-evaluation of your own continuing professional development.

a Are you a member of an EBM-style journal club?

b Have you participated in or tutored at one of the workshops on how to practice or teach EBM?

c Have you joined the evidence-based-health e-mail discussion group?

d Have you established links with other practitioners or teachers of EBM?

[1] If so, please share them with the developers of this course!

[2] If so, please add them to the bank of EBCH educational resources that the Centre for Evidence-based Child Health shared with other educators around the world.

Glossary of terms you are likely to encounter in your clinical reading

This glossary is intended to provide guidance as to the meanings of terms you will come across frequently in clinical articles, especially when they appear in EBM journals.

Absolute risk reduction (ARR) – *see* ***Treatment effects***

Case-control study – a study which involves identifying patients who have the outcome of interest (cases) and control patients without the same outcome, and looking back to see if they had the exposure of interest (*see also* ***Review of study designs***).

Case-series – a report on a series of patients with an outcome of interest. No control group is involved.

Clinical practice guideline – is a systematically developed statement designed to assist practitioner and patient decisions about appropriate health care for specific clinical circumstances.

Cohort study – involves identification of two groups (cohorts) of patients, one which did receive the exposure of interest, and one which did not, and following these cohorts forward for the outcome of interest (*see also* ***Review of study designs***).

Confidence interval (CI) – the range within which we would expect the true value of a statistical measure to lie. The CI is usually accompanied by a percentage value which shows the level of confidence that the true value lies within this range. For example, for an NNT of 10 with a 95% CI of 5 to 15, we would have 95% confidence that the true NNT value was between 5 and 15.

Control event rate (CER) – *see* ***Treatment effects***.

Cost-benefit analysis – assesses whether the cost of an intervention is worth the benefit by measuring both in the same units; monetary units are usually used.

Cost-effectiveness analysis – measures the net cost of providing a service as well as the outcomes obtained. Outcomes are reported in a single unit of measurement.

Cost-minimisation analysis – if health effects are known to be equal, only costs are analysed and the least costly alternative is shown.

Cost-utility analysis – converts effects into personal preferences (or utilities) and describes how much it costs for some additional quality gain (e.g. cost per additional quality-adjusted life-year, or QALY).

Crossover study design – the administration of two or more experimental therapies one after the other in a specified or random order to the same group of patients (*see also* ***Review of study designs***).

Cross-sectional study – the observation of a defined population at a single point in time or time interval. Exposure and outcome are determined simultaneously (*see also* ***Review of study designs***).

Decision analysis – is the application of explicit, quantitative methods that quantify prognoses, treatment effects, and patient values in order to analyse a decision under conditions of uncertainty.

Ecological survey – a survey based on aggregated data for some population as it exists at some point or points in time; to investigate the relationship of an exposure to a known or presumed risk factor for a specified outcome.

Event rate – the proportion of patients in a group in whom the event is observed. Thus, if out of 100 patients, the event is observed in 27, the event rate is 0.27. Control event rate (CER) and experimental event rate (EER) are used to refer to this in control and experimental groups of patients respectively. The patient expected event rate (PEER) refers to the rate of events we'd expect in a patient who received no treatment or conventional treatment – *see* ***Treatment effects***.

Evidence-based health care – extends the application of the principles of evidence-based medicine (*see* below) to all professions associated with health care, including purchasing and management.

Evidence-based medicine – the conscientious, explicit and judicious use of current best evidence in making decisions about the care of individual patients. The practice of evidence-based medicine means integrating individual clinical expertise with the best available external clinical evidence from systematic research. *See also* Sackett *et al.* (1996) EBM: What it is and what it isn't. *BMJ* **312:** 71–2.

Experimental event rate (EER) – *see* ***Treatment effects***.

Incidence – the proportion of new cases of the target disorder in the population at risk during a specified time interval.

Inception cohort – a group of patients assembled near the onset of the target disorder.

Intention to treat analysis – a method of analysis for randomised trials in which all patients randomly assigned to one of the treatments are analysed together, regardless of whether or not they completed or received that treatment.

Likelihood ratio (LR) – the likelihood that a given test result would be expected in a patient with the target disorder compared to the likelihood that that same result would be expected in a patient without the target disorder.

Calculation of sensitivity/specificity/LR:

	DISEASE POSITIVE	DISEASE NEGATIVE
TEST POSITIVE	a	b
TEST NEGATIVE	c	d

Sensitivity = a/(a+c)

$$\text{LR+} = \frac{\text{sensitivity}}{\text{1-specificity}} = \frac{a/(a+c)}{b/(b+d)}$$

Specificity = d/(b+d)

$$\text{LR–} = \frac{\text{(1-sensitivity)}}{\text{specificity}} = \frac{c/(a+c)}{d/(b+d)}$$

Positive predictive value = a/(a+b)   Negative predictive value = d/(c+d)

Meta-analysis – is a systematic review that uses quantitative methods to summarise the results.

N-of-1 trials – in such trials, the patient undergoes pairs of treatment periods organised so that one period involves the use of the experimental treatment and one period involves the use of an alternate or placebo therapy. The patients and physician are blinded, if possible, and outcomes are monitored. Treatment periods are replicated until the clinician and patient are convinced that the treatments are definitely different or definitely not different.

Negative predictive value – proportion of people with a negative test who are free of the target disorder (*see also* ***Likelihood ratio***).

Number needed to treat (NNT) – is the inverse of the absolute risk reduction and is the number of patients that need to be treated to prevent one bad outcome – *see* ***Treatment effects***.

Odds – a ratio of non-events to events. If the event rate for a disease is 0.1 (10%), its non-event rate is 0.9 and therefore its odds are 9:1. Note that this is not the same expression as the inverse of event rate.

Odds ratio (OR) – is the odds of having the target disorder in the experimental group relative to the odds in favour of having the target disorder in the control group (in prospective case-control studies, overviews) or the odds in favour of being exposed in subjects with the target disorder divided by the odds in favour of being exposed in control subjects (without the target disorder).

Calculations of OR/RR for use of trimethoprim-sulfamethoxazole prophylaxis in cirrhosis:

	Adverse event occurs (infectious complication)	Adverse event does not occur (no infectious complication)	Totals
Exposed to treatment (experimental)	1 a	29 b	30 a+b
Not exposed to treatment (control)	c 9	d 21	c+d 30
Totals	a+c 10	b+d 50	a+b+c+d 60

CER = c/(c+d) = 0.30
EER = a/(a+b) = 0.033
Control Event Odds = c/d = 0.43
Experimental Event Odds = a/b = 0.034
Relative Risk = EER/CER = 0.11
Relative Odds = Odds Ratio = (a/b)/(c/d) = ad/bc = 0.08
Patient expected event rate – *see* ***Treatment effects***.

Overview – *see* ***systematic review.***

Positive predictive value – proportion of people with a positive test who have the target disorder (*see also* ***Likelihood ratio***).

Post-test odds – the odds that the patient has the target disorder after the test has been carried out (pre-test odds and likelihood ratio).

Post-test probability – The proportion of patients with that particular test result who have the target disorder.

Pre-test odds – the odds that the patient has the target disorder before the test has been carried out (pre-test probability / 1–pre-test probability).

Pre-test probability/prevalence – the proportion of people with the target disorder in the population at risk at a specific time or time interval.

Randomised controlled clinical trial (RCT) – a group of patients is randomised into an experimental group and a control group. These groups are followed up for the variables / outcomes of interest (*see also* ***Review of study designs***).

Relative risk reduction (RRR) – *see* ***Treatment effects***.

Risk ratio (RR) – is the ratio of risk in the treated group (EER) to the risk in the control group (CER) – used in randomised trials and cohort studies:

RR = ERR/CER

Sensitivity – proportion of people with the target disorder who have a positive test. It is used to assist in assessing and selecting a diagnostic test/sign/symptom (*see also* ***Likelihood ratio***).

SnNout – when a sign/test/symptom has a high **S**ensitivity, a **N**egative result rules **out** the diagnosis, e.g. the sensitivity of a history of ankle swelling for diagnosing ascites is 93%, therefore if a person does not have a history of ankle swelling, it is highly unlikely that the person has ascites.

Specificity – proportion of people without the target disorder who have a negative test. It is used to assist in assessing and selecting a diagnostic test/sign/symptom (*see also* ***Likelihood ratio***).

SpPin – when a sign/test/symptom has a high **S**pecificity, a **P**ositive result rules **in** the diagnosis, e.g. the specificity of a fluid wave for diagnosing ascites is 92%, therefore if a person does have a fluid wave, it rules in the diagnosis of ascites.

Systematic review – *a summary of the medical literature that uses explicit methods to perform a thorough literature search and critical appraisal of individual studies, and that uses appropriate statistical techniques to combine these valid studies.*

Treatment effects

The E-B journals have achieved consensus on some terms they use to describe both the good and the bad effects of therapy. They will join the terms already in current use (RRR, ARR, NNT), and both sets are described here and summarised in the Glossary that appears inside the back cover of *Evidence-based Medicine*. We will bring them to life with a synthesis of three randomised trials in diabetes which individually showed that several years of intensive insulin therapy reduced the proportion of patients with worsening retinopathy to 13% from 38%, raised the proportion of patients with satisfactory haemoglobin A1c levels to 60% from about 30%, and increased the proportion of patients with at least one episode of symptomatic hypoglycaemia to 47% from 23%. Note that in each case the first number constitutes the 'experimental event rate' or EER and the second number the 'control event rate' or CER. We will use the following terms and calculations to describe these effects of treatment:

When the experimental treatment reduces the probability of a bad outcome (worsening diabetic retinopathy).

RRR (Relative risk reduction): the proportional reduction in rates of bad outcomes between experimental and control participants in a trial, calculated as |EER – CER|/CER, and accompanied by a 95% confidence interval (CI). In the case of worsening diabetic retinopathy, |EE – CER|/CER = |13% – 38%|/38% = 66%.

ARR (Absolute risk reduction): the absolute arithmetic difference in rates of bad outcomes between experimental and control participants in a trial, calculated as |EER – CER|, and accompanied by a 95% CI. In this case, |EER – CER| = |13% – 38%| = 25%.

NNT (Number needed to treat): the number of patients who need to be treated to achieve 1 additional favourable outcome, calculated as 1/ARR and accompanied by a 95% CI. In this case, 1/ARR = 1/25% = 4.

Calculations for the occurrence of diabetic retinopathy in IDDMs:

Occurrence of diabetic neuropathy at 5 yr among insulin-dependent diabetics in the DCCT trial		**Relative risk reduction (RRR)**	**Absolute risk reduction (ARR)**	**Number needed to treat (NNT)**
Usual insulin regimen CER	Intensive insulin regimen EER	$\frac{\lvert EER - CER \rvert}{CER}$	$\lvert EER - CER \rvert$	1/ARR
13%	38%	$\frac{\lvert 13\% - 38\% \rvert}{38\%} = 66\%$	$\lvert 13\% - 38\% \rvert = 25\%$	1/25% = 4 pts, for 6 years, with intensive insulin Rx

When the experimental treatment increases the probability of a good outcome (satisfactory haemoglobin A1c levels).

RBI (Relative benefit increase): the proportional increase in rates of good outcomes between experimental and control patients in a trial, calculated as |EER-CER|/CER, and accompanied by a 95% confidence interval (CI). In the case of satisfactory haemoglobin A1c levels, |EER – CER|/CER = |60% – 30%|/30% = 100%.

ABI (Absolute benefit increase): the absolute arithmetic difference in rates of good outcomes between experimental and control patients in a trial, calculated as |EER – CER|, and accompanied by a 95% CI. In the case of satisfactory haemoglobin A1c levels, |EER – CER| = |60% – 30%| = 30%.

NNT (Number needed to treat): The number of patients who need to be treated to achieve one additional good outcome, calculated as 1/ARR and accompanied by a 95% CI. In this case, 1/ARR = 1/30% = 3.

When the experimental treatment increase the probability of a bad outcome (episodes of hypoglycaemia).

RRI (Relative risk increase): the proportional increase in rates of bad outcomes between experimental and control patients in a trial, calculated as |EER – CER|/CER, and accompanied by a 95% CI. In the case of hypoglycaemic episodes, |EER – CER|/CER = |57% – 23%|/57% = 34%/57% = 60%. (RRI is also used in assessing the impact of 'risk factors' for disease.)

ARI (Absolute risk increase): the absolute arithmetic difference in rates of bad outcomes between experimental and control patients in a trial, calculated as |EER – CER|, and accompanied by a 95% CI. In the case of hypoglycaemic episodes, |EER – CER| = |57% – 23%| = 34%. (ARI is also used in assessing the impact of 'risk factors' for disease.)

NNH (Number needed to harm): the number of patients who, if they received the experimental treatment, would lead to one additional patient being harmed, compared with patients who received the control treatment, calculated as 1/ARR and accompanied by a 95% CI. In this case, 1/ARR = 1/34% = 3.

		Adverse Outcome		Totals
		Present (case)	**Absent (control)**	
Exposed to the Treatment	Yes (cohort)	a	b	a+b
	No (cohort)	c	d	c+d
	Totals	a+c	b+d	a+b+c+d

In a randomised trial or cohort study:
Relative risk = RR = [a/(a+b)]/[c/(c+d)]

In a case-control study:
Odds ratio (or Relative odds) = OR = ad/bc

Randomized controlled trial: start with a+b+c+d and randomise to (a+b) and (c+d)

Advantages

1 Assignment to treatment can be kept concealed.

2 Confounders equally distributed.

3 Blinding more likely.

4 Randomisation facilitates statistical analysis.

Disadvantages

1 Expensive – time and money.

2 Volunteer bias.

3 Ethically problematic at times.

Crossover design

Advantages

1 Subjects serve as own controls and error variance is reduced thus reducing sample size needed.

2 All subjects receive treatment (at least some of the time).

3 Statistical tests assuming randomisation can be used.

4 Blinding can be maintained.

Disadvantages

1 All subjects receive placebo or alternative treatment at some point.

2 Washout period lengthy or unknown.

3 Cannot be used for treatments with permanent effects.

Cohort study: selects (a+b) and (c+d)

Advantages

1 Ethically safe.

2 Subjects can be matched.

3 Can establish timing and directionality of events.

4 Eligibility criteria and outcome assessments can be standardised.

5 Administratively easier and cheaper than RCT.

Disadvantages

1 Controls may be difficult to identify.

2 Exposure may be linked to a hidden confounder.

3 Blinding difficult.

4 Still expensive.

5 Randomisation not present.

6 For rare disease, large sample sizes or long follow-up necessary.

Cross-sectional (analytic) survey: selecting a+b+c+d

Advantages

1 Cheap and simple.

2 Safe ethically.

Disadvantages

1 Establishes association at most, not causality.

2 Recall bias susceptibility.

3 Confounders may be unequally distributed.

4 Neyman bias.

5 Group sizes may be unequal.

Case-control study: selecting (a+c) and (b+d)

Advantages

1 Quick and cheap.

2 Only feasible method for very rare disorders or those with long lag between exposure and outcome.

3 Fewer subjects needed than cross-sectional studies.

Disadvantages

1 Reliance on recall or records to determine exposure status.

2 Confounders.

3 Selection of control groups difficult.

4 Potential bias – recall, selection.

Section 3a1

Is this evidence about a diagnostic test valid?

Having found a possibly useful article about a diagnostic test, how can you quickly critically appraise it for its proximity to the truth? This can be done by asking some simple questions; often you'll find their answers in the article's abstract. Table 3a1.1 lists these questions for individual reports, but you can also apply them to the interpretation of a systematic review (overview) of several different studies of the same diagnostic test for the same target disorder.*

The first guide is: 'Was there an independent, blind comparison with a reference ("gold") standard of diagnosis?' This is quite a mouthful, but it simply means that two criteria should have been met. The patients in the study should have undergone *both* the diagnostic test in question (say, an item of the history or physical examination, a blood test, etc.) *and* the reference (or 'gold') standard (an autopsy or biopsy or other confirmatory 'proof' that they do or don't have the target disorder); and the results of one shouldn't be known to those who are applying and interpreting the other (for example, the pathologist interpreting the biopsy that comprises the reference standard for the target disorder should be 'blind' to the result of the blood test that comprises the diagnostic test under study). In this way, investigators avoid the conscious and unconscious bias that otherwise might cause the reference standard to be 'overinterpreted' when the diagnostic test is positive and 'underinterpreted' when it is negative. Sometimes investigators have a difficult time coming up with clearcut

* As we'll stress throughout this book, systematic reviews will give you the most valid and useful external evidence on just about any clinical question you can pose. They are still pretty rare for diagnostic tests and for this reason we'll describe them in their usual, therapeutic habitat, in Section 3a3. When using Table 3a3.2 to consider diagnostic tests, simply substitute 'diagnostic test' for 'treatment' as you read.

Table 3a1.1 Are the results of this diagnostic study valid?

1. **Was there an independent, blind comparison with a reference ('gold') standard of diagnosis?**
2. **Was the diagnostic test evaluated in an appropriate spectrum of patients (like those in whom it would be used in practice)?**
3. **Was the reference standard applied regardless of the diagnostic test result?**

reference standards (e.g. for psychiatric disorders) and you'll want to give careful consideration to their arguments justifying the selection of their reference standard.

One way or another, the report will wind up calling some results 'normal' and others 'abnormal' and we'll show you how to interpret these in Section 3b1. For now, you might simply want to recognize that there are six definitions of 'normal' in common use (we've listed them in Table 3a1.2). We will make use of definition 5 ('diagnostic' normal) and believe that half of the definitions are not useful. The first two (the Gaussian and percentile definitions) are derived from the study test results alone, with no reference standard, and simply define the 'normal range' for the diagnostic test result on the basis of statistical properties (standard deviations or percentiles). Thus they are properties of the test in isolation from any objective reality. These don't make any sense to us, for they imply that all 'abnormalities' occur at the same frequency. They both suggest that if we can perform enough diagnostic tests on a patient we are bound to find something 'abnormal' and lead to all sorts of inappropriate further testing. The third definition of 'normal' (culturally desirable) represents a cultural value judgment . It is seen in fashion advertisements and at the fringes of the 'lifestyle' movement where medicine becomes confused with morality. The fourth (risk factor) definition has the drawback that it 'labels' or stigmatizes some patients and is clinically useful only if we can do something positive to lower their risk. The fifth (diagnostic) definition is the one that we will focus on here and we will show you how to generate and interpret diagnostic normality in Section 3b1. The final (therapeutic) definition is in part an outgrowth of the

Table 3a1.2 Six definitions of normal

1. **Gaussian: the mean +/– 2 standard deviations. Assumes a normal distribution and means that all 'abnormalities' have the same frequency.**
2. **Percentile: within the range, say, of 5–95%. Has the same basic defect as the Gaussian definition.**
3. **Culturally desirable: preferred by society. Confuses the role of medicine.**
4. **Risk factor: carrying no additional risk of disease. Labels the outliers, who may not be helped.**
5. **Diagnostic: range of results beyond which target disorders become highly probable – the focus of this discussion.**
6. **Therapeutic: range of results beyond which treatment does more good than harm. Means you have to keep up with advances in therapy!**

fourth (risk factor) definition and has the great clinical advantage that it changes with our knowledge of efficacy. Thus, the definition of normal blood pressure has changed radically over the past few decades as we have learned that treatment of progressively lower blood pressure levels does more good than harm.

Returning to the second question in Table 3a1.1, you will want the diagnostic test to have been evaluated in an appropriate spectrum of patients, similar to the practice population in which the test might be used. Among patients with late or severe disease, when the diagnosis is obvious, often you won't need any diagnostic test, so studies that confine themselves to florid cases are not very informative. The article will be informative if the diagnostic test was applied to patients with mild as well as severe and early as well as late cases of the target disorder and among both treated and untreated individuals. In addition, you would want the diagnostic test to have been applied to patients with different disorders that are commonly confused with the target disorder of interest.

Finally, was the reference standard applied regardless of the diagnostic test result? When patients have a negative diagnostic test result, investigators are tempted to forego applying the reference standard and when the latter is invasive or risky (e.g. angiography) it may be considered inappropriate to do so. For this reason, many investigators now employ a reference standard for a patient *not* having the target disorder in which they *don't* suffer any adverse health outcome during a long follow-up on no definitive treatment (for example, convincing evidence that a patient with clinically suspected deep vein thrombosis did *not* have this disorder would be a prolonged follow-up on no antithrombotic therapy and suffering no ill effects).

If the report you're reading fails one or more of these three tests you'll need to consider whether it has a fatal flaw that renders its conclusions invalid; if so, it's back to more searching (either now or later; if you haven't enough time, perhaps you can interest a colleague or trainee in taking this on). If the report passes this initial scrutiny and you decide that you can believe its results, but you haven't already carried out the second critical appraisal step of deciding whether these results are impressive, then you can proceed to Section 3b1 on page 118.

Further reading

Jaeschke R, Guyatt G H, Sackett D L for the Evidence-Based Medicine Working Group. Users' guides to the medical literature. VI. How to use an article about a diagnostic test. A: Are the results of the study valid? JAMA 1994; 271: 389–91.

Section 3a2

Is this evidence about prognosis valid?

Clinicians consider questions about prognosis all the time. Sometimes the questions are posed by patients and are quite direct (How long have I got?). At other times the questions are posed by clinicians and are indirect, as when deciding *whether* to treat at all (e.g. an elderly man with chronic lymphocyte leukemia who feels well – would his prognosis be importantly altered if he were left alone until he becomes symptomatic?) or deciding *whether* to screen (e.g. for abdominal aortic aneurysms – what is the fate of the undetected 4 cm aneurysm?). These questions share two elements: a qualitative aspect (Which outcomes could happen?) and a temporal aspect (Over what time period?). In Chapter 1 we showed you how to recognize such questions as being about prognosis and in Chapter 2 we addressed how to find good information about prognosis. In this part of Chapter 3 we'll present a framework for appraising the validity and importance of evidence about prognosis, for use when you tackle situations like the ones above (see Table 3a2.1). We'll consider them in sequence.

The four guides that will help you decide whether some evidence about prognosis is valid are listed in Table 3a2.1. First of all, was a defined, representative sample of patients assembled at a common (usually early) point in the course of their disease? Ideally, the prognosis study you find would include the entire population of patients who ever lived who developed the disease, studied from the instant of its onset. Since this is impossible, you'll want to look at how far from ideal will still tell you what you need to know and you'll do that by finding the methods section (if there isn't one, maybe you're wasting your time on this report!) and reading how the study patients were assembled. You'd want their illness to be defined well enough for you to be clear about it and you'd want the entire spectrum of severity that would occur at that common point to be represented.

Table 3a2.1 Is this evidence about prognosis valid?

1. Was a defined, representative sample of patients assembled at a common (usually early) point in the course of their disease?
2. Was patient follow-up sufficiently long and complete?
3. Were objective outcome criteria applied in a 'blind' fashion?
4. If subgroups with different prognoses are identified:
   - Was there adjustment for important prognostic factors?
   - Was there validation in an independent group of 'test-set' patients?

But when should the 'clock start'? That is, from what point in the disease should patients be followed? If investigators begin tracking outcomes only *after* several patients have already finished their course with the disease, then the outcomes for these patients would never be counted. Some would have recovered quickly, whilst others might have died quickly. So, to avoid missing outcomes by 'starting the clock' too late, you should look to see that study patients were included at a uniformly early time in the disease, ideally when it first becomes clinically manifest, the so-called 'inception cohort'. An exception might be if you wanted to learn about the prognosis of a late stage in the disease (e.g. for clinically manifest coronary heart disease); in this case you'd look for a representative and well-defined sample of patients who were all at a similarly advanced stage (e.g. when they had their first clinical coronary event, not when they first developed elevated coronary risk factors).

Second, was patient follow-up sufficiently long and complete? Ideally, every patient in the inception cohort would be followed over time until they fully recover or one of the disease outcomes occurs. If with short follow-up few study patients have any of the outcomes of interest, you won't have enough to go on when advising your patients. Of course, if after decades of follow-up few adverse events have occurred, this good prognostic result is very useful in reassuring your patient about the future. If you think that the follow-up is too short to have developed a valid picture of the extent of the outcome of your interest, you'd better look for other evidence.

If follow-up was long enough, you still have to worry about patients who entered the study but got lost along the way. Patients are almost always lost to follow-up and their outcomes will be excluded from the study's conclusions about prognosis. Some losses to follow-up are both unavoidable and unrelated to prognosis (e.g. moving away to a better job) and these aren't a cause for worry. But other losses might be because patients die or are too ill to continue follow-up (or lose their independence and move in with family) and the failure to document and report their outcomes will threaten the validity of the report. Short of finding a report that kept track of every patient, how can you judge whether follow-up is 'sufficiently complete'? There is no single answer for all studies, but we offer two suggestions to help you make this judgment. The first is a simple '5 and 20' rule of thumb: fewer than 5% loss probably leads to little bias, greater than 20% loss seriously threatens validity and in-between amounts cause intermediate amounts of trouble. While this may be easy to remember, it may oversimplify for clinical situations in which the outcomes are infrequent.

The second approach uses a 'worst-case' scenario. Imagine a study of prognosis wherein 100 patients enter the study, four die and 16 are lost to follow-up. A 'crude' survival rate would count the four deaths among the 84 with total follow-up, for a death rate of 4.8%, and then report a survival rate of 100% – 4.8% = 95.2%. But what of the lost 16? Some or all of them might have died too. The latter, 'worst-case' scenario would mean a case-fatality rate of (four known + 16 lost) or 20 out of (84 followed up + 16 lost) or 20/100, that is 20% (four times the observed rate!); note that in order to determine the 'worst-case' scenario you've added the lost patients to both the numerator and denominator of the outcome rate. On the other hand, in the 'best-case' scenario none of the lost 16 would have died, yielding a case-fatality rate of 4 out of (84 + 16) or 4/100, that is 4%; note that in determining the 'best-case' scenario you add the missing cases to just the denominator. While this 'best case' of 4% may not differ much from the observed 4.8%, the 'worst case' of 20% does differ meaningfully and you'd probably judge that this study's follow-up

was not sufficiently complete. By seeing what effect the losses might have on the result you can decide whether a 'worst-case' scenario would change your conclusion about prognosis. If this simple form of 'sensitivity analysis' suggests that losses wouldn't change the result much, then you can judge the follow-up as sufficiently complete.

You can use these first two guides to screen articles about prognosis to find the few worth more of your limited time. If you've answered 'no' to both of the above questions, you can be pretty sure the study will not provide estimates of prognosis that are close to the truth and you ought to start searching for better evidence. If, on the other hand, you've answered 'yes' to both of the above questions, you can be reasonably confident that the study will provide accurate information about prognosis. To be even more sure of this, you should ask the remaining two validity questions in Table 3a2.1.

Were objective outcome criteria applied in a 'blind' fashion? Diseases can affect patients in many important ways; some are easy to spot and some are more subtle. In general, outcomes at both extremes, death or full recovery, are relatively easy to detect and be sure of. In between these extremes are a wide range of outcomes that can be more difficult to detect or confirm and where investigators will have to use judgment in deciding how to count them up. Examples include the degree of disease activity/quiescence, the readiness for return to work and the intensity of residual pain. To minimize the effects of bias, investigators can establish specific criteria that define each possible outcome of the disease and then use these criteria during patient follow-up. You can usually find such outcome criteria in the text, tables, appendices or references in the study. You should satisfy yourself that they are sufficiently objective for confirming the outcomes you're interested in. The occurrence of death is about as objective as you can get, but judging the underlying cause of death is very prone to error (especially when it's based on death certificates) and can be biased unless objective criteria are applied to high-quality clinical evidence.

But even with objective criteria, some bias might creep in if the investigators judging the outcomes also know the

patients' characteristics. To minimize this bias, the authors of the report should have taken precautions so that the investigators making judgments about clinical outcomes were 'blind' to these patients' clinical characteristics and prognostic factors. The more subjective the outcome, the more important such blinding becomes. You should satisfy yourself that blinding was used if it would have been important for the outcomes of interest to you.

The final pair of guides have to do with reports that claim that one subgroup of patients has a different prognosis from others. Such reports are common and for good clinical reason. Often you will want to know whether subgroups of patients have different prognoses (e.g. among patients with non-valvular atrial fibrillation, are those with enlarged left atria at higher risk for stroke than those with normal sized atria?). The first guide here suggests that you look to see whether there was adjustment for other important prognostic factors. That is, reports that address this sort of question should have made sure that these subgroup predictions aren't being distorted by the unequal occurrence of another, powerful prognostic factor (such as would occur if patients with large atria were also more likely to have had prior embolic stroke than patients with normal atria). There are both simple (e.g. stratified analyses displaying the prognoses of patients with large atria separately for those with and without prior embolic stroke) and fancy (e.g. multiple regression analyses that could take into account not only prior embolic stroke but also hypertension, left ventricular function and the like) ways of adjusting for these other important prognostic factors and you should reassure yourself that one or the other has been applied before you tentatively accept the conclusion about a different prognosis for the subgroup of interest.

We say tentatively because there is one final guide to deciding whether a claim that a subgroup has a different prognosis should be accepted as valid. This is the fact that the statistics of determining subgroup prognoses are all about prediction, not explanation. They are indifferent to whether the prognostic factor is physiologically logical (in our running example, left atrial size) or biologically nonsensical (whether the patient's navel is concave (an 'innie') or convex (an 'outie')). These prognostic factors can be demographic (such as age, gender, socioeconomic status), disease specific (such as extent of disease, degree of test abnormality) or comorbid (presence or absence of many other conditions). Keep in mind that these prognostic factors need not cause the outcome; they need only be associated with its development strongly enough to predict it.

For this reason, the first time a prognostic factor is identified, there is no guarantee it isn't the result of a random, non-causal 'quirk' in its distribution between patients with different prognoses; for that reason, the initial patient group in which it was identified is called a 'training set'. As you might imagine, if this initial study carried out a multivariate analysis looking for potential prognostic factors, they'd be very likely to find at least a few, just on the basis of chance (and most investigators would be imaginative enough to suggest logical explanations for them). Because of this risk of spurious, chance nomination of prognostic factors, you should seek its confirmation in a report of a second, independent group (called a 'test set') of patients. The best evidence for this is finding a statement (in the methods section) of a prestudy intention to examine this specific possible prognostic factor (based on its appearance in a training set). If that second, independent study also identifies the prognostic factor, you can feel much more confident that the evidence about it is valid.

If your evidence flunks these tests for validity, we're afraid it's back to searching, either now (if you still have time) or at a later session. If, on a happier note, you decide that the evidence you've found about a prognostic factor is valid and you haven't already decided whether it's also important, you can take that consideration up in Section 3b2 on page 129.

Further reading

Laupacis A, Wells G, Richardson W S, Tugwell P for the Evidence-Based Medicine Working Group. Users' guides to the medical literature. V. How to use an article about prognosis. JAMA 1994; 272: 234–7.

Section 3a3

Is this evidence about a treatment valid?

Having found some possibly useful evidence about therapy, you have to decide where to start in its critical appraisal. On the one hand, you could start here in Section 3a3, with an appraisal of its validity (arguing that if it's not valid, who cares whether it appears to show a big effect?). On the other, you could go right to determining its importance in Section 3b3 (arguing that if the evidence doesn't suggest a possibly useful clinical impact, who cares if it's valid?). Begin with either and then pick up the other. This section will help you to quickly and critically appraise evidence about therapy for its closeness to the truth. This can be done by asking some simple questions and often you'll find their answers in an abstract that accompanies the evidence. Table 3a3.1 lists these questions for reports of individual therapeutic trials, but since these can best be interpreted in the context of all other trials on the same topic, Table 3a3.2 summarizes guides for assessing evidence that has combined the results of several trials into an overview or systematic review (when a systematic review uses special statistical methods for combining the results of several studies, we call it a meta-analysis). Alternatively, you may encounter (or have tracked down) an economic analysis, which is a more complex method that compares therapeutic alternatives from a broader perspective (including those of health managers or even society as a whole) and tries to offer or provide treatments in the way that best uses scarce resources such as hospital beds, drugs, operating time, clinicians and money. Questions pertinent to deciding whether you should believe an economic analysis appear in Table 3a3.3. Finally, and building on the earlier section on diagnosis, we'll give you a brief description of how to decide whether to believe evidence on the effects of therapy when it is formulated into a clinical decision analysis; rules for deciding whether to believe their results are described in Section 3a3.4.

Table 3a3.1 Are the results of this single study valid?

The main questions to answer:

1. **Was the assignment of patients to treatments randomized? and was the randomization list concealed?**
2. **Were all patients who entered the trial accounted for at its conclusion? and were they analyzed in the groups to which they were randomized?**

And some finer points to address:

1. **Were patients and clinicians kept 'blind' to which treatment was being received?**
2. **Aside from the experimental treatment, were the groups treated equally?**
3. **Were the groups similar at the start of the trial?**

When several randomized trials of the same treatment for the same condition have been carried out, we think you'll agree that an overview which systematically reviews and combines all of them would give you a better answer than a critical appraisal of just one of them. For that reason, we suggested back in Chapter 2 that you always start your search for useful clinical articles on just about any topic by looking for systematic reviews. However, because systematic reviews assess their component trials individually (and, as you can see in Table 3a3.2, you want to be sure that they've done that in a valid way) and since at this point in history you're much more likely to find individual trials than systematic reviews, we'll begin with the individual trial.

Is the evidence from this randomized trial valid?

We'll begin with two important questions:

1. Was the assignment of patients to treatments randomized and was the randomization schedule concealed?

When deciding whether the evidence from a randomized trial is valid, the most important question to ask (and frequently the quickest question to answer) is: Was the assignment of patients to treatments randomized? That is, was some method analogous to tossing a coin* used to assign patients to treatments (with the treatment you're interested in given if the coin landed 'heads' and a conventional, 'control' or placebo† treatment given if the coin landed 'tails')? The reason for insisting on random allocation to treatments is that this comes closer than any other research design to creating groups of patients at the start of the trial who are identical in their risk of the events you're hoping to prevent. It does this in two, related ways. First, the coin toss balances the groups for prognostic factors (such as disease severity or other predictors of especially good or bad prognosis) which, if they were unevenly distributed between treatment groups, could exaggerate, cancel or even counteract the effects of therapy.‡ If they exaggerated the apparent effects of an otherwise ineffectual treatment, the effects of their imbalance could lead to the false-positive conclusion that the treatment was useful when it was not. And if they cancelled or counteracted the effects of a really efficacious treatment, the effects of their imbalance could lead to the false-negative conclusions that a useful treatment was useless or even harmful. Random allocation balances the treatment groups for these and other prognostic factors, even if we don't yet understand the disorder well enough to know what they are!

The second, related benefit of random allocation is that, if it is concealed from the clinicians who are entering patients into the trial, they will be unaware of which treatment the next patient will receive and they can't either consciously or unconsciously distort the balance between the groups being compared. So you want to be sure that both of these standards are met. Usually it's easy to tell whether a study was

* In practice, this coin tossing is done by special computer programs, but the principle is exactly the same.
† A placebo is a treatment that is so similar in appearance, taste, etc. that the patient ('single-blind') or the clinician or both ('double-blind') are unable to distinguish it from the active treatment.
‡ 'Confounder' is a technical name for these sorts of patient characteristics that are extraneous to the question posed, could cause the clinical events we are trying to prevent with the treatment and might be unevenly distributed between the treatment groups. And although there are other ways of avoiding confounding (exclusion, stratified sampling, matching, stratified analysis, standardization and multivariate modelling), they all demand that you already know what the confounder is.

randomized, because it's something to be proud of and that term often appears in the title and almost always in the abstract. On the other hand, it's not often stated whether the randomization list was concealed, but if randomization occurred by telephone or by some system that was at a distance from where patients were being entered into the trial, you can be comfortable about this. If randomization wasn't concealed, this tends to lead to patients with more favourable prognoses being given the experimental treatment, exaggerating the apparent benefits of therapy and perhaps even leading to the false-positive conclusion that the treatment is efficacious when it is not.

If you find that the study was not randomized, we'd suggest that you stop reading it and go on to the next article. Only if you can't find any randomized trials should you come back and have another go at it. But if the only evidence you have about a treatment is from non-randomized studies, you are in a bind and have five options:

1. Check Chapter 2 again or get help in doing another literature search to see if you missed any randomized trials of the candidate therapy.
2. See whether the treatment effect is simply so huge that you can't imagine it could be a false-positive study (this usually happens only when the prognosis is uniformly awful and is a very rare situation). As a check, ask several colleagues whether they consider the candidate therapy so likely to be efficacious that they'd consider it unethical to randomize a patient like yours into a study of it that includes a no-treatment or placebo group.*
3. Conversely, if the non-randomized study concluded that the treatment was useless or harmful, then it is usually safe to accept that conclusion (since, as described above, false-negative conclusions from non-randomized studies are less likely than false-positive ones).
4. Consider whether an 'N-of-1' trial would make sense to you and your patient (they are described on page 173).

* This is the 'convincing non-experimental evidence' category used in the audits of clinical care reported on page 3 (the A-team study).

5. Try some other treatment or simply provide supportive care.

2. Were all patients who entered the trial accounted for at its conclusion and were they analysed in the groups to which they were randomized?

Having satisfied yourself that the trial really was randomized, you can then match the number of patients who entered the trial with the number accounted for at its conclusion. Ideally, these numbers will be identical, for lost patients could have had events that would change the conclusion. If, for example, patients on the experimental treatment dropped out and had adverse outcomes, their absence from the analysis would lead it to overestimate the efficacy of that treatment. What's an acceptable loss? To be sure of a trial's conclusion, its authors should be able to take all patients who were lost along the way, assign them the 'worst-case' outcomes (that is, assume that everyone lost from the group whose remaining members fared better had a bad outcome and assume that everyone lost from the group whose remaining members fared worse had a rosy outcome) and still be able to support their original conclusion. It would be unusual for a trial to withstand a worst-case analysis if it lost more than 20% of its patients and journals like *Evidence-Based Medicine* won't publish trials with <80% follow-up.

Because anything that happens after randomization can affect the chances that a patient in a trial has an event, it's important that all patients (even those who fail to take their medicine or accidentally or intentionally receive the wrong treatment) are analysed in the groups to which they were randomized. This is an essential prerequisite for valid evidence about the effects of therapy. For example, it has repeatedly been shown that patients who do and don't take their study medicine have very different outcomes, even when the study medicine they have been prescribed is a placebo! The correct form of analysis, in which patients are analysed in the groups to which they were assigned, is called an 'intention to treat' analysis.

There are three less important questions to ask when you are trying to decide whether a randomized trial has produced valid evidence:

1. Were patients and clinicians kept 'blind' to which treatment was being received?
2. Aside from the experimental treatment, were the groups treated equally?
3. Were the groups similar at the start of the trial?

If you decide that the study really was randomized, follow-up was virtually complete and patients were analyzed in the groups to which they'd been randomized, you can look for some other features that provide even greater assurance that you can believe its results. If, for example, it was a pharmacological trial in which patients received either a tablet containing the active drug or an identical-appearing (in size, shape, colour, taste, etc.) tablet of pharmacologically inert ingredients (a placebo), then it would be possible to keep both patients and clinicians blind* as to which treatment was received and neither the patient's reporting of symptoms nor the clinician's interpretation of them would be influenced by their hunches about whether the treatment was efficacious. Another advantage of the double-blind method is that it prevents patients and their clinicians from adding any additional treatments (or 'cointerventions') to just one of the groups. When patients and their clinicians can't be kept blind (as in surgical trials), often it is possible to have other, blinded clinicians come in and assess clinical records (purged of any mention of treatment) or make special outcome measurements. And finally, you can double-check to see whether randomization was effective by looking to see whether patients were similar at the start of the trial (most trials display this in the first table of their results).

Whether the results of an individual trial are important is considered in Section 3b3 on page 133.

* When patients don't know their treatment but their doctors do (as when the active drug causes a clearcut sign such as bradycardia), the trial is called 'single blind'. When both are blind, it is called 'double blind'.

Is the evidence from this systematic review valid?

Having shown you how to decide whether to believe the results of a single trial, let's now turn to how you can decide whether to believe the results of an overview of several trials. The key questions you need to answer are in Table 3a3.2.

Table 3a3.2 Are the results of this systematic review valid?

1. Is it an overview of randomized trials of the treatment you're interested in?
2. Does it include a methods section that describes:
a. finding and including all the relevant trials?
b. assessing their individual validity?
3. Were the results consistent from study to study?

1. Is it a systematic review of randomized trials of the treatment you're interested in?

This first question asks whether you are sure that the treatment is the same as the one you're considering and immediately asking whether the overview is combining reports of studies carried out at the same, most powerful level of evidence that we've been discussing here, the randomized trial. Systematic reviews of non-randomized studies of therapy simply compound the problems of individually misleading trials and the same warnings apply. Moreover, some overviews combine randomized and non-randomized studies and unless the authors have provided separate information on the subset of randomized trials, you shouldn't trust them either.

2. Does it include a methods section that describes: (a) finding and including all the relevant trials; (b) assessing their individual validity?

You should see whether the overview report includes a methods section that describes how they found all the relevant trials and how they assessed their individual validity. Let's take these three elements one by one. First, because performing an overview is performing research (it involves posing a question, identifying a population and drawing a sample, making measurements, analyzing them and drawing

conclusions), it should be carried out and reported like research. If you don't find a methods section, be very wary of believing its results; maybe its only useful part will be its bibliography of individual trials for you to study as above. Second, if the overview has a methods section it should describe how its authors tracked down and included all the trials that were relevant to this treatment. This is no easy task. The standard bibliographic databases described in Chapter 2, good as they are, fail to correctly label up to half of the published trials and 'negative' trials (that conclude the treatment is not efficacious) are less likely to be submitted for publication, leading an overview of those that are published to overestimate the treatment's efficacy. Signs that the overviewers did a good job are positive when they report at least some hand searching of the most relevant journals (for miscoded trials) and especially when they report contacting the authors of published trials (who often will know about unpublished ones). Third, you should look for a statement of how they decided whether the individual trials in their overview were scientifically sound, using criteria like those in Table 3a3.1. Finally, because these last two steps of deciding which trials to include in the overview involve a lot of judgment calls, you should be especially reassured when you find that two or more investigators carried out these tasks independent of each other and achieved good agreement about their judgments.

3. Were the results consistent from study to study?

It stands to reason that we are more likely to believe an overview when the results of all the trials in it show a treatment effect going in the same direction. Although we shouldn't expect each of them to show exactly the same degree of efficacy (that is, we should be comfortable with a certain amount of quantitative difference in the trial results), we would be concerned if we found some trials in an overview confidently concluding a beneficial effect of the treatment and other trials confidently concluding no benefit or a harmful effect. Such a qualitative difference in the effects of treatment (which also goes by the name of heterogeneity), unless it can be explained to your satisfaction (such as by differences in patients or in doses or durations of treatment), should lead you to be very cautious about believing any overall conclusion about efficacy in all patients and you'd hope to see your caution expressed in the conclusions of the overview.

Whether the results of an overview are important is considered in Section 3b3 on page 133.

Section 3a4

Is this evidence about harm valid?

You must frequently make judgments on whether a treatment is harming or has harmed a patient. Many admissions to acute general hospitals are the result of adverse drug reactions and reactions to diagnostic and therapeutic maneuvers are judged to befall one-fifth to one-third of patients after they are admitted. On the other hand, even clinical pharmacologists disagree about whether a given patient has had an adverse drug reaction and the fact that an adverse reaction occurred *during* a treatment is insufficient evidence that it occurred *because* of that treatment.

Faced with a problem that is pandemic yet controvertible, clinicians must equip themselves to answer two related questions:

1. Does this drug (or operation or other treatment) cause that adverse effect in *some* patients? And, if so:
2. Did this drug (or operation or other treatment) cause that adverse effect in *this particular* patient?

This section will deal with the first question and the second question will be addressed in Section 4.4.

Because this assessment can be viewed as addressing a general question of *causation*, it benefits from what has been learned about asking and answering such questions in classical epidemiology. The four guides for deciding whether to believe the claim that a treatment harms some patients are summarized in Table 3a4.1, and we'll consider them in sequence.

1. Were there clearly defined groups of patients, similar in all important ways other than exposure to the treatment?

Because the 'threats to validity' are different for different sorts of studies, you'll have to spend just a little time sorting them out. Suppose you wanted to decide whether fenoterol (a beta-agonist used to treat asthma) sometimes (albeit

Table 3a4.1 Are the results of this harm study valid?

1. Were there clearly defined groups of patients, similar in all important ways other than exposure to the treatment?
2. Were treatment exposures and clinical outcomes measured in the same way in both groups?
3. Was the follow-up of study patients complete and long enough?
4. Do the results satisfy some 'diagnostic tests for causation'?
- Is it clear that the exposure preceded the onset of the outcome?
- Is there a dose-response gradient?
- Is there positive evidence from a 'dechallenge–rechallenge' study?
- Is the association consistent from study to study?
- Does the association make biological sense?

rarely) caused the death of its users. You could look for and find four different sorts of studies and all of them can be illustrated by reference to Table 3a4.2. First, you could look for a randomized trial in which asthma patients were assigned, by a system analogous to tossing a coin, to receive fenoterol (the top row in Table 3a4.2, whose total is **a+b**)

		Adverse Outcome		Totals
		Present (Case)	Absent (Control)	
Exposed to the treatment	Yes (Cohort)	a	b	a+b
	No (Cohort)	c	d	c+d
	Totals	a+c	b+d	a+b+c+d

Table 3a4.2 Different ways of finding out whether a treatment sometimes causes harm or some comparison treatment or placebo (the bottom row, whose total is **c+d**). Since the randomization would make them similar for all other features that would cause their deaths, you'd be pretty likely to judge any statistically significant increase in deaths among fenoterol recipients (cell **a**) as valid. Trouble is, if fenoterol causes only one extra death per 1000 users, you'd have to find an awfully big trial to show a clear excess among fenoterol-treated asthmatics. As it happens, if a drug causes an adverse reaction once per x patients who receive it (say, once per 1000), to be 95% certain to see at least one adverse reaction you need to follow 3x patients (in this example, 3000). For that reason, you usually can't find the most valid data on harm from individual randomized trials and if you can't find a systematic review with a large enough total number of patients to suffice, you'll have to work with non-experimental evidence.

The next most powerful design is also conducted along the rows of Table 3a4.2, but this time the groups of patients (called 'cohorts') who are (**a+b**) and are not (**c+d**) exposed to the treatment are formed not by random allocation, but by the decisions of clinicians and patients to have some of them ('exposed') receive the treatment and others ('unexposed') not receive it. These cohorts are then followed to determine which and how many of them develop the bad outcome (**a** or **c**). As you can see, there is no reason why these cohorts should be otherwise perfectly identical to each other and plenty of reason for them to be quite different (e.g. sicker patients who are more likely to have adverse outcomes might be more likely to be offered a 'last-ditch' treatment). Since there may be strong links between the prognosis of patients and the probability that they will be offered and accept a treatment (sometimes called 'confounding'), the analyses of these cohort analytic studies are difficult and often involve trying to correct for known confounders (such as disease severity) by statistical methods (all the way from simply comparing outcomes within patients with different degrees of severity to quite fancy multivariate analyses). But we can't adjust for what we don't yet know about the determinants of disease outcomes, so you have to be cautious in interpreting cohort studies.

And for rare or late complications of treatments, not even cohort studies are big enough and often you'll have to rely on studies conducted vertically in Table 3a4.2 by assembling cases (**a+c**) who already have the bad outcome, assembling a second group of 'controls' (**b+d**) who don't have the bad outcome and tracking back in their histories or records to determine the proportions of each group who were exposed to the suspect treatment (**a** or **b**): a case-control study. This is, in fact, what was done in trying to sort out the fenoterol problem: asthma deaths (cases) were compared with living asthma patients (controls) for their use of fenoterol and these comparisons were 'adjusted' for the severity of their asthma. The problem of confounding (of prognosis with exposure) is even worse in case-control studies than in cohort studies, for often it is impossible to measure the confounders among cases, even if they are known.* For this reason, case-control studies are viewed with even greater caution than cohort studies. Finally, you may find reports of one or a few patients who developed the bad outcome while under treatment (just cell **a**). If the outcome is unique and dramatic (phocomelia in children born to women who took thalidomide) case reports and case series may be enough, but usually they simply point to the need for the other types of studies.

As with other issues in clinical and health care, the best evidence on adverse effects will come from a systematic review of all the relevant studies and these should always be your primary targets when searching for the best external evidence. Systematic reviews of randomized trials or cohort studies may possess sufficiently large numbers of patients to identify even rare adverse effects. Whether appraising a systematic review or an individual study, you'll need to take into account how it assembled and assessed its members and now that you've learned how to recognize the sort of study you're reading, you can apply the guides in Table 3a4.1:

1. From the foregoing discussion, it's clear why you want the report to describe clearly defined groups of

* Dead patients tell no tales and information about exposures to lethal treatments may perish with their victims.

patients, similar in all important ways other than exposure to the treatment (to get rid of confounders).

2. Moreover, it makes sense that you should place greater confidence in reports of studies in which treatment exposures and clinical outcomes were measured the same ways in both groups (you'd not want one group studied more exhaustively than the other, because this would lead to reporting a greater occurrence of exposure or outcome in the more intensively studied group).

3. Furthermore, in a report concluding that the treatment was innocent, you'd want the follow-up of study patients to have been complete and long enough for the bad effects to have had time to reveal themselves.

4. Finally, you'd want to determine whether the association met at least some common-sense 'diagnostic tests for causation':

- you'd want to be sure that the exposure (say, use of a psychotropic drug) preceded the onset of the bad outcome (say, behavior ending in suicide), and wasn't just a 'marker' (say, of depression) that it was already underway;
- the validity of a claim that a treatment causes an adverse outcome receives a real boost when increasing doses or durations of the treatment are associated with increasing frequency or severity of the adverse outcome: a 'dose–response' effect;
- the validity of a claim is also boosted if there is documentation that the adverse effect decreased or disappeared when the treatment was withdrawn ('dechallenge') and worsened or reappeared when the treatment was reintroduced ('rechallenge');
- if you are fortunate enough to have found a systematic review of the question, you can determine whether the association of exposure to the suspect treatment and the adverse outcome is consistent from study to study. When it is, your confidence in the validity of the association deserves to increase;
- finally, it boosts your confidence when the association makes biological sense.

If the report fails to meet the first three minimum standards, you're better off abandoning it and continuing your search. On the other hand, if you're satisfied that the report meets these minimum guides, you can decide whether the relation between exposure and outcome is strong and convincing enough for you to need to do something about it and that's discussed in Section 3b4.

Further reading

Levine M, Walter S D, Lee H, Haines T, Holbrook A, Moyer V for the Evidence-Based Medicine Working Group. Users' guides to the medical literature: IV. How to use an article about harm. JAMA 1994; 271: 1615–19.

Section 3b1

Is this evidence about a diagnostic test important?

In deciding whether the evidence about a diagnostic test is important, we will focus on a modern way of thinking about diagnosis that takes into account both components of evidence-based medicine: your individual clinical expertise and the best external evidence. The former is your prior assessment of diagnostic possibilities before you do the test ('prior or pretest probabilities') and the latter is the ability of the test to distinguish patients with and without the target disorder (both the oldfashioned concepts of sensitivity and specificity and the newfangled and more powerful ideas around likelihood ratios). We'll show you how to combine these two elements of EBM to refine your estimates of the target disorder ('posterior or post-test probabilities') and make the diagnosis. Diagnostic tests that produce big changes from pretest to post-test probabilities are important and likely to be useful to you in your practice.

Where do these pretest probabilities come from? Usually they are derived from your own accumulating clinical experience, specific for the setting in which you work and the sorts of patients you see. As a result, pretest probabilities for the same target disorder can vary widely between and within countries and between primary, secondary and tertiary care. We have summarized some published pretest probabilities in Table 3b1.1 and more are available from our Website.

Suppose that you're working up a patient with anemia and think that the probability that they have iron deficiency anemia is 50%; that is, the odds are about 50–50 that it's due to iron deficiency. When you present the patient to your boss, you ask for an educational prescription to determine the usefulness of performing a serum ferritin on your patient as a means of detecting iron deficiency anemia. Suppose further that, in filling your prescription, you find a systematic

Table 3b1.1 Some pretest probabilities

Patient problem	Clinical setting	Target disorder	Pretest probability
Melena in a 50-year-old man who drinks 25 units of alcohol a week but has no stigmata of liver disease	Emergency room in North America	Varices	5%
		Benign ulcer	55%
		Gastritis	40%
Symptomless 60–69-year-olds	Primary care	Undiagnosed colon cancer: all patients	0.5%
		positive family history	1.5%
Symptomless	Primary care	≥ 75% stenosis of one or more coronary arteries	
Woman 30–39 y/o			0.3%
60–69 y/o			8%
Man	30–39 y/o		2%
	60–69 y/o		12%
Non-anginal chest pain			
Woman 30–39 y/o			1%
60–69 y/o			19%
Man 30–39 y/o			5%
60–69 y/o			28%
Atypical angina			
Woman 30–39 y/o			4%
60–69 y/o			54%
Man 30–39 y/o			22%
60–69 y/o			67%
Typical angina pectoris			
Woman 30–39 y/o			26%
60–69 y/o			91%
Man 30–39 y/o			70%
60–69 y/o			94%
Symptomless 50 y/o with a solitary pulmonary nodule	Primary care	Cancer	
		for any nodules	50%
		For 3 cm nodules	65%

To find more examples, and to nominate additions to the databank of pretest probabilities, refer to this textbook's Website at: http://cebm.jr2.ox.ac.uk/

review of several studies of this diagnostic test (evaluated against the reference standard of a bone marrow stain for iron), decide that it is valid (based on the guides in Tables 3a3.2 and 3a1.1), and find their results as shown in Table 3b1.2. By the time you've tracked down and studied the external evidence, your patient's serum ferritin comes back at 60 mmol/L. How should you put all this together?

As you can see from Table 3b1.2, your patient's result places them in the top row of the table, either in cell **a** or cell **b**. From that fact you would conclude several things: first, you'd note that 90% of patients with iron deficiency have serum ferritins in the same range as your patient, (**a/(a+c)**, and that property, the proportion of patients with the target disorder who have positive test results, is called sensitivity.

Table 3b1.2 Results of a systematic review of serum ferritin as a diagnostic test for iron deficiency anemia

		Target disorder (iron deficiency anemia)		Totals
		Present	Absent	
Diagnostic test result (serum ferritin)	Positive (<65 mmol/L	731 a	270 b	1001 a+b
	Negative (≥65 mmol/L	78 c	1500 d	1578 c+d
	Totals	809 a+c	1770 b+d	2579 a+b+c+d

Sensitivity = **a/(a+c)** = 731/809 = 90%
Specificity = **d/(b+d)** = 1500/1770 = 85%
LR+ = sens/(1−spec) = 90%/15% = 6
LR− = (1−sens)/spec = 10%/85% = 0.12
Positive predictive value = **a/(a+b)** = 731/1001 = 73%
Negative predictive value = **d/(c+d)** = 1500/1578 = 95%
Prevalence = **(a+c)/(a+b+c+d)** = 809/2579 = 32%
Pretest odds = prevalence/(1−prevalence) = 31%/69% = 0.45
Post-test odds = pretest odds × likelihood ratio
Post-test probability = post-test odds/(post-test odds +1)

And you might also note that only 15% of patients with other causes for their anemia have results in the same range as your patient,* which means that your patient's result would be about six times as likely (90% / 15%) to be seen in someone with, as opposed to someone without, iron deficiency anemia and that's called the likelihood ratio for a positive test result. Furthermore, since you thought ahead of time (before you had the result of the serum ferritin) that your patient's odds of iron deficiency were 50–50, that's called a pretest odds of 1:1 and, as you can see from the formulae towards the bottom of Table 3b1.2, you can multiply that pretest odds of 1 by the likelihood ratio of 6 to get the post-test odds of iron deficiency anemia after the test: 1×6 = 6. Since, like most clinicians, you may be more comfortable thinking in terms of probabilities than odds, this post-test odds of 6:1 converts (as you can see at the bottom of Table 3b1.2) to a post-test probability of 6/(6+1) = 6/7 = 86%. So it looks like you've made the diagnosis and this diagnostic test looks worthwhile.

(To check yourself out on these calculations, try the same ferritin result for a patient who, like those in the table, has a pretest odds of 0.47;† you'll know you did it right if you wind up with an answer identical to its equivalent, the positive predictive value.)

Extremely high values of sensitivity and specificity are useful, but not for the reasons you may think.‡ When a test has a very high sensitivity (such as the loss of retinal vein pulsation in increased intracranial pressure), a negative result (the presence of pulsation) effectively rules out the diagnosis (of raised intracranial pressure) and one of our clinical clerks suggested that we apply the mnemonic SnNout to such findings (when a sign has a high *Sen*sitivity, a *N*egative result

* The complement of this proportion is called specificity and it describes the proportion of patients who do not have the target disorder who have negative or normal test results, **d/(b+d)**.
† The post-test odds are 0.45 × 6 = 2.7 and the post-test probability is 2.7/3.7 = 73%. Note that this is identical to the positive predictive value.
‡ On first encounter, most learners think that tests with high sensitivity rule in diagnoses and tests with high specificity rule them out; the reverse is the case.

rules *out* the diagnosis). Similarly, when a sign has a very high specificity (such as a fluid wave for ascites), a positive result effectively rules in the diagnosis (of ascites); not surprisingly, our clinical clerks call such a finding a SpPin (when a sign has a high *Sp*ecificity, a *P*ositive result rules *in* the diagnosis). We've listed some SpPins and SnNouts in Table 3b1.3 and have generated a longer list on our Website.

Although the serum ferritin determination looks impressive when viewed in terms of its sensitivity (90%) and specificity (85%), the newer way of expressing its accuracy with likelihood ratios reveals its even greater power and, in this particular example, shows how we can be misled by the fact that the old sensitivity–specificity approach restricts us to just two levels (positive and negative) of the test result. Most test results, like serum ferritin, can be divided into several levels and in Table 3b1.4 we show you a particularly useful way of dividing test results into five levels. When this is done, one extreme level of the test result can be shown to rule in the diagnosis and in this case you can SpPin 59% of the patients with iron deficiency anemia, despite the unimpressive sensitivity (59%) that would have been achieved if the ferritin results had been split at this level. Likelihood ratios of 10 or more, when applied to pretest probabilities of 33% or more (.33/.67 = pretest odds of 0.5) will generate post-test probabilities of 5/6 = 83% or more. Moreover, the other extreme level can SnNout 75% of those who do not have iron deficiency anemia (again despite a not very impressive specificity of 75%). Likelihood ratios of 0.1 or less, when applied to pretest probabilities of 33% or less (.33/.67 = pretest odds of 0.5) will generate post-test probabilities of 0.05/1.05 = 5% or less. Two other intermediate levels can move a 50% prior probability (pretest odds of 1:1) to the useful but not usually diagnostic post-test probabilities of 4.8/5.8 = 83% and 0.39/1.39 = 28%. And one indeterminate level in the middle (containing about 10% of both sorts of patients) can be seen to be uninformative, with a likelihood ratio of 1. We've shown the effects of these sorts of likelihood ratios on these sorts of pretest probabilities in Table 3b1.5.

Table 3b1.3 Some SpPins and SnNouts

Target disorder	SpPin (& specificity) [presence rules in the target disorder]	SnNout (& sensitivity) [absence rules out the target disorder]
Ascites (by imaging or tap)*	Fluid wave (92%)	History of ankle swelling (93%)
Pleural effusion†	Auscultatory percussion note loud and sharp (100%)	Auscultatory percussion note soft and/or dull (96%)
Increased intracranial pressure (by CAT scan or direct measurement)‡		Loss of spontaneous retinal vein pulsation (100%)
Cancer as a cause of lower back pain (by further investigation)§		Age >50 or cancer history or unexplained weight loss or failure of conservative therapy (100%)
Sinusitis (by further investigation)¶		Maxillary toothache or purulent nasal secretion or poor response to nasal decongestants or abnormal transillumination or history of coloured nasal discharge
Alcohol abuse or dependency**	Yes to ≥3 of the CAGE questions (99.8%)	
Splenomegaly (by imaging)††	Positive percussion (Nixon method) and palpation	
Non-urgent cause for dizziness‡‡	Positive head-hanging test and either vertigo or vomiting (94%)	

To find more examples, and to nominate additions to the databank of SpPins and SnNouts, refer to this textbook's Website at: http://cebm.jr2.ox.ac.uk/

* JAMA 1992; 267: 2645–8.
† J Gen Int Med 1994; 9: 71–4.
‡ Arch Neurol 1978; 35: 37–40.
§ JAMA 1992; 268: 760–5.
¶ JAMA 1993; 270: 1242–6.
** Amer J Med 1987; 82: 231–5.
†† JAMA 1993; 270: 2218–21.
‡‡ JAMA 1994; 271: 385–8.

Table 3b1.4 The usefulness of five levels of a diagnostic test result

Diagnostic test result	Serum ferritin (mmol/L)	Target disorder present: Number	Target disorder present: %	Target disorder absent: Number	Target disorder absent: %	Likelihood ratio	Diagnostic impact
Very positive	<15	474	59%	20	1.1%	52	Rule in SpPin
Moderately positive	15–34	175	22%	79	4.5%	4.8	Intermediate high
Neutral	35–64	82	10%	171	10%	1	Indeterminate
Moderately negative	65–94	30	3.7%	168	9.5%	0.39	Intermediate low
Extremely negative	≥95	48	5.9%	1332	75%	0.08	Rule out SnNout
		809	100%	1770	100%		

Table 3b1.5 Some post-test probabilities generated by five levels of a diagnostic test result

Likelihood ratio	Post-test probability of the target disorder for different pretest probabilities: Pre-test 5%	Pre-test 10%	Pre-test 20%	Pre-test 30%	Pre-test 50%	Pre-test 70%	Diagnostic impact
Very positive 10	34%	53%	71%	81%	91%	96%	Rule in SpPin
Moderately positive 3	14%	25%	43%	56%	75%	88%	Intermediate high
Neutral 1	5%	10%	20%	30%	50%	70%	Indeterminate
Moderately negative 0.3	1.5%	3.2%	7%	11%	23%	41%	Intermediate low
Extremely negative 0.1	0.5%	1%	2.5%	4%	9%	19%	Rule out SnNout

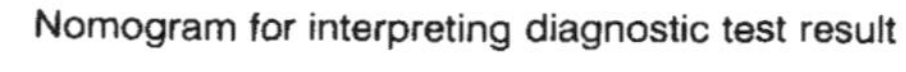

Finally, there's an easier way of manipulating all these probability↔odds calculations and a nomogram for doing so appears as Figure 3b1.1 and in the pocket cards that come with this book. You can check out your understanding of this nomogram by replicating the results in Table 3b1.5.

To your surprise (we reckon!) your patient's test result generates an indeterminate likelihood ratio of only 1 and the test which you thought might be very useful, based on the sensitivity and specificity way of looking at things, really hasn't been helpful in moving you toward the diagnosis, so you'll have to think about other tests (including perhaps the reference standard of a bone marrow examination) to sort this out.

More and more reports of diagnostic tests are providing multilevel likelihood ratios as measures of their accuracy. When they only report sensitivity and specificity, you can sometimes find a table with more levels and generate your own set of likelihood ratios or you can find a scatter plot (of test results versus diagnoses) that is good enough for you to be able to split into levels. Or, if all you have is sensitivity and specificity, you can generate likelihood ratios from them by reference to the formulae in Table 3b1.2 (the likelihood ratio for a positive test result = LR+ = sensitivity/[1-specificity] and the likelihood ratio for a negative test result = LR− = [1-sensitivity]/specificity).

Some reports into the accuracy of diagnostic tests go beyond even likelihood ratios and one of them deserves mention here. This extension considers multiple diagnostic tests as a cluster or sequence of tests for a given target disorder. These multiple results can be presented in different ways, either as clusters of positive/negative results or as multivariate scores, and in either case they can be ranked and handled just like other multilevel likelihood ratios.

In any event, having decided that a diagnostic test produces important changes from pretest to post-test probabilities, you might want to study the final issue, described in Section 4.1, of how to integrate the results of this critical appraisal with your individual clinical expertise and apply the results

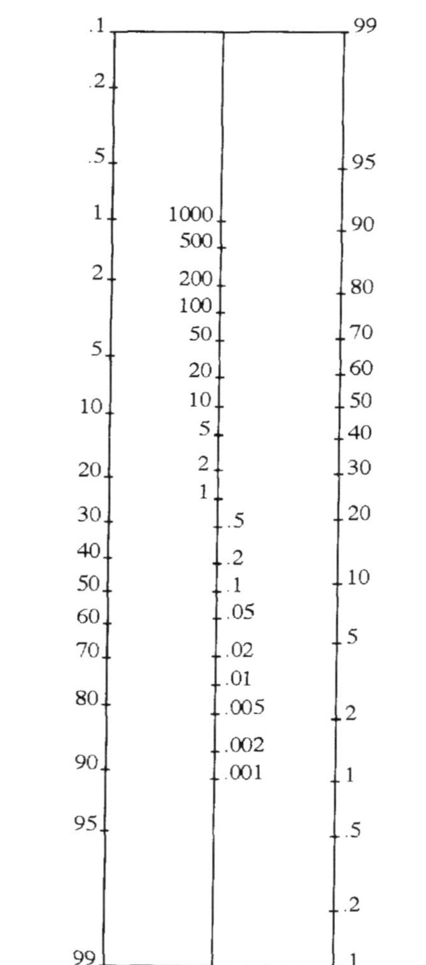

Figure 3b1.1 A likelihood ratio nomogram. Adapted from Fagan T J 1975 Nomogram for Bayes's Theorem (c). New England Journal of Medicine 293: 257

to your own patient (but if you jumped to this second step without first determining whether the evidence about this diagnostic test was valid, you'd better go back to Section 3a1 first!).

Further reading

Sackett D L, Haynes R B, Guyatt G H, Tugwell P. Clinical epidemiology: a basic science for clinical medicine, 2nd edn. Little, Brown, Boston, 1991. Chapter 4 (for interpreting diagnostic tests).

Jaeschke R, Guyatt G H, Sackett D L for the Evidence-Based Medicine Working Group. Users' guides to the medical literature. VI. How to use an article about a diagnostic test. A. Are the results of the study valid? JAMA 1994; 271: 389–91. B. What are the results and will they help me in caring for my patients? JAMA 1994; 271: 703–7.

Section 3b2

Is this evidence about prognosis important?

Guides for making this decision appear in Table 3b2.1. First, how likely are the outcomes over time? Diseases usually have more than a single outcome of interest and these can occur in several combinations and at different times following the onset of the disease. Thus, for each important disease outcome, you should examine the article to see how likely each of these outcomes is over time. Typically they are reported as percentage survival at a particular point in time (such as 1-year or 5-year survival rates) and as survival curves of various kinds. Another form of result, common in cancer studies, is the median survival, indicating the length of follow-up by which 50% of the study sample have died. The more numerous the outcome possibilities and the more variable the timing of these outcomes are, the more complex such results can be.

Figure 3b2.1 illustrates some different patterns of prognosis, each leading to different conclusions about prognosis. They are presented in the most frequent format used to describe prognosis, a survival curve that depicts, at each point in time, the proportion (often expressed as a %) of the original study population who have NOT yet had an outcome event.* In panel A, virtually no patients have had events by the end of the study, so either the prognosis is very good (in which case the study is very useful to you) or the study is too short (in which case it's not very useful!). Panels B, C and D depict a serious disease, with only

* How such survival curves are constructed is not described in detail in this book, so don't look for it! In brief, it is done by some clever methods that combine the results from patients who have been followed for just short periods of time as well as long ones and who have had outcomes occur early, late or not at all. Often the strategy used here is a 'life table' method, if you want to look it up.

Table 3b2.1 Is this evidence about prognosis important?

1. How likely are the outcomes over time?
2. How precise are the prognostic estimates?

20% of patients surviving at 1 year; you could tell such patients, then, that their chances of surviving for a year are 20%. Note, however, that the shapes of these curves are quite different, so that the median survival (by which time half of them have succumbed) is 9 months for the disorder described in panel B but only 3 months for the disorder described in panel C. The survival pattern is a steady, uniform decline only in panel D and we hope you can see why the best answer to 'How much time have I got, doc?' often is the time at which half the study patients have died (or suffered some other event of interest); this is called the median survival.

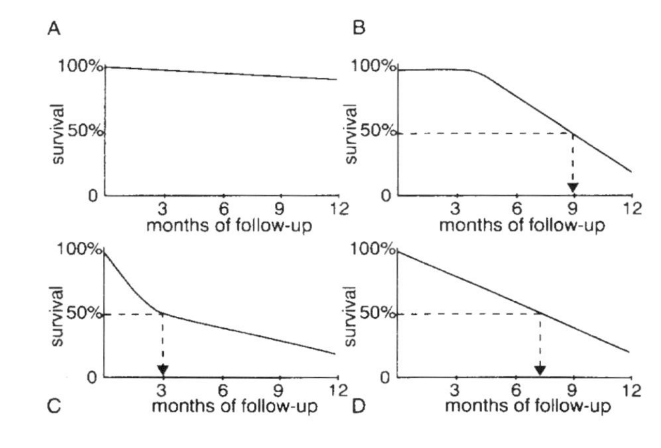

Figure 3b2.1 Prognosis shown as survival curves. Panel A: Good prognosis (or too short a study!). Panel B: Good prognosis early, then worsening, with a median survival of 9 months. Panel C: Bad prognosis early, then better, with a median survival of 3 months. Panel D: Steady prognosis, with a median survival of 6 months

The second guide asks you to consider how precise the prognostic statements are. As we mentioned in Section 3a2, investigators study prognosis in a sample of diseased patients, not in the whole population of everyone who has ever had the disease. Purely by the play of chance, then, the identical study done 100 times over with different samples from that same whole population would yield differing results. In deciding whether these prognostic results are important, then, you will need some means of judging just how much these results could vary by chance alone, that is, the precision of the results. This is best done with the 95% confidence interval:* in those 100 repetitions of the identical study with different samples, 95 would be within a calculable distance of the true prognosis (some lower and some higher). For example, an article on the prognosis of first strokes among 675 patients reported a case-fatality rate of 20% in the first month, with the 95% confidence interval of 17–23%; that interval is pretty narrow and if the report was valid, it looks important as well. If, on the other hand, that 20% was based on just 20 patients, the 95% confidence interval on death in the first month would run from 2% to 38% and that is so wide (almost 20-fold) that you couldn't regard the result as important and potentially useful to you. The text, tables or graphs should tell you the confidence interval for the prognosis and you can decide whether it is too big for you to trust it.

That completes your critical appraisal of evidence about prognosis. If you decide that the evidence you've found is both valid and important, you could go to Section 2 of Chapter 4 (page 164) and decide whether and how to apply it to your patient.

* We describe the confidence interval in the Appendix. In this case, the confidence interval on a prognosis (expressed as a decimal) is the observed result plus or minus 1.96 times the square root of {[(the observed result) × (1 – the observed result)] / sample size}. So, for the original study 20% = 0.2 and the confidence interval becomes 0.2 +/– 1.96 times the square root of {[(0.2) × (0.8)]/675} or 0.2 +/– 0.03 or 17–23%. As a check on your understanding, you can see if you can calculate the confidence interval when the sample is just 40 stroke patients.

Further reading

Laupacis A, Wells G, Richardson W S, Tugwell P for the Evidence-Based Medicine Working Group. Users' guides to the medical literature. V. How to use an article about prognosis. JAMA 1994; 272: 234–7.

Section 3b3

Is this evidence about a treatment important?

This section will help you determine the size and potential benefits of the effects of the treatment described in a report, whether you've decided (from the previous section) that the report is valid or whether you start here. Because our primary perspective in this book is the individual clinician, the main measure we will show you how to develop and use is the number of patients a clinician needs to treat in order to prevent one additional adverse outcome (NNT) and along the way we will show you both the absolute risk reduction (ARR) and relative risk reduction (RRR) in the occurrence of adverse outcomes achieved by active therapy. We'll also introduce you to the bare bones of assessing the results of an economic analysis, a more complex method that we employ in determining the effects of therapy when we are taking the broader perspective (usually in collaboration with health managers) of deciding how groups of patients, or society as a whole, should be provided or offered treatments in the way that best uses scarce resources such as hospital beds, drugs, operating time, clinicians and money. Finally, we'll give you a brief description of how evidence on the effects of therapy can be formulated into a clinical decision analysis.

In Section 3 of Chapter 4, we'll show you how to extrapolate the measures from each of these three approaches to individual patients, in order to answer the question: Can I apply these results to my patient?

Is the evidence from this randomized trial important?

Introducing some measures of the effects of therapy

Knowing whether you should be impressed with the results of a valid therapeutic trial requires two steps: first, finding the

most useful clinical expression of these results (or converting data from the report into this most useful expression); and second, comparing those results with the results of other treatments for other conditions. We'll take these one at a time.

The relative risk reduction (RRR)

The Diabetes Control and Complications Trial into the effect of intensive diabetes therapy on the development and progression of neuropathy, which we've summarized in Table 3b3.1, confirmed neuropathy occurred among 9.6% of patients randomized to usual care (1–2 insulin injections/day to prevent glycemic symptoms; we'll call that the control event rate or CER) and 2.8% (we'll call that the experimental event rate or EER) among patients randomized to intensive therapy (insulin pump or =>3 injections per day).

This difference was statistically highly significant, but how might this treatment effect be expressed in terms of its clinical significance? The traditional measure of this effect is the proportional or 'relative' risk reduction (abbreviated RRR in our journal), calculated as (CER–EER)/CER. In this example, the RRR is (9.6% – 2.8%) / 9.6% or 71%; intensive therapy reduced the risk of developing neuropathy by 71%.

Why not confine our description of the clinical significance of this result to the relative risk reduction (RRR)? The reason is that the RRR fails to discriminate huge absolute treatment effects (10 times those observed in this trial) from trivial ones (one ten-thousandth of those observed here). For example, if the rates of neuropathy were 10 times those observed in this trial (the 'high hypothetical case' in Table 3b3.1), and a whopping 96% of control patients and 28% of intensively treated patients developed neuropathy, the relative risk reduction would remain unchanged: RRR = (96% – 28%) / 96% or 71%. And if a trivial 0.00096% of control and 0.00028% of intensively treated patients developed neuropathy (the 'low hypothetical case' in Table 3b3.1), the

Table 3b3.1 Clinically useful measures of the effects of treatment

The occurrence of neuropathy	Event rates (diabetic neuropathy)		Relative risk reduction	Absolute risk reduction	Number needed to be treated (to prevent one event)
	Usual insulin regimen (CER)	Intensive insulin regimen (EER)	RRR = $\frac{\text{CER–EER}}{\text{CER}}$	ARR = (CER–EER)	NNT = 1/ARR
In the actual trial	9.6%	2.8%	$\frac{9.6\% - 2.8\%}{9.6\%} = 71\%$	9.6% – 2.8% = 6.8%	$\frac{1}{6.8\%} = 14.7$ or 15
High hypothetical case A	96%	28%	$\frac{96\% - 28\%}{96\%} = 71\%$	(96% – 28%) = 68%	$\frac{1}{68\%} = 1.47$ or 2
Low hypothetical case B	0.00096%	0.00028%	$\frac{(0.00096\% - 0.00028\%)}{0.00096\%} = 71\%$	(0.00096% –0.00028%) = 0.00068%	$\frac{1}{0.00068\%} = 147\,000$

relative risk reduction is as before: RRR still = (0.00096% – 0.00028%) / 0.00096 = 71%! This is because the relative risk reduction discards the underlying susceptibility (or 'baseline risk') of patients entering randomized trials; as a result, the relative risk reduction cannot discriminate huge risks and benefits from small ones.

The absolute risk reduction (ARR)

In contrast to these non-discriminating relative risk reductions, the absolute difference in the rates of neuropathy between control and experimental patients (CER–EER) clearly does discriminate between these extremes and this measure is called the absolute risk reduction or ARR. In the trial, the ARR or (CER–EER) = 9.6% – 2.8% = 6.8%; in the high hypothetical case, where 96% of control patients and 28% of intensively treated patients developed neuropathy, the ARR = 96% – 28% = 68% and in the low hypothetical case in which a trivial 0.00096% of control and 0.00028% of intensively treated patients developed neuropathy, the ARR = 0.00096% – 0.00028% = 0.00068%. These absolute risk reductions retain the underlying susceptibility of patients and provide more complete information than relative risk reductions. And when treatment increases the occurrence of some good event (rather than decreasing the occurrence of some bad event) we can generate an absolute risk increase or ARI. But, unlike relative risk reductions (RRRs), absolute risk reductions and increases (ARRs and ARIs) are difficult to remember and don't slip easily off the tongue at the bedside (lots of clinicians become queasy with numbers less than 1.0).

The number of patients that need to be treated (NNT) to prevent one bad outcome

If, however, we divide the absolute risk reduction into 1 (that is, if we 'invert' the ARR or 'take its reciprocal' so that it becomes 1/ARR), we generate a very useful number, for it represents the number of patients we need to treat (NNT)

with the experimental therapy in order to prevent one of them from developing the bad outcome.* In this case, we would generate the number of diabetics we would need to treat with the intensive regimen in order to prevent one of them from developing neuropathy. In the trial, the NNT is 1/ARR or 1/6.8% or 14.7; we usually round that number upwards (in this case, to 15) and we now can say that for every 15 patients who are treated with the more intensive insulin regimen, one will be prevented from developing diabetic neuropathy.

Is this a large or a small number of patients that need to be treated to prevent one bad outcome? Now we're ready to pursue that second step in deciding whether to be impressed with the valid results of a therapeutic trial. Like many important matters in medicine, the answer has to do with clinical significance, not statistical significance. This NNT of 15 certainly is far smaller than the number of patients we'd need to treat in the extremely low hypothetical example, in which 1/ARR becomes 1/(0.00068%) or an NNT of more than 147 000, a figure so vast that we can't imagine anyone judging that it was worth the effort. We can get a better idea by comparing this NNT of 15 with that for other interventions we are familiar with in medicine.

In doing so, we add the additional dimension of the duration of therapy: in the diabetes trial treatment went on for an average of 6.5 years, meaning that we need to treat about 15 diabetics for about 6.5 years with an intensive insulin regimen to prevent one of them from developing neuropathy. How does this compare with other treatments, over other durations, for other conditions? We show some of them (with the event rates appearing as decimals rather than percents) in Table 3b3.2. Beginning on an optimistic note, we need to treat only about 20 chest pain patients who appear to be having heart attacks with streptokinase and aspirin to save a life at 5 weeks. On the other hand, we need to treat about 70 elderly hypertensives for 5 years with antihypertensive drugs

* Similarly, 1/ARI tells us how many individuals we need to treat to cause one additional good outcome.

Table 3b3.2 Some NNTs for different treatments

Condition or disorder	Intervention	Events being prevented	Event Rates: Control Event Rate CER	Event Rates: Experimental Event Rate EER	Duration of follow-up	NNT to prevent one additional event
Diabetes (IDDM)*	Intensive insulin regimens	Diabetic neuropathy	0.096	0.028	6.5 years	15
Diabetes (NIDDM)†	Intensive insulin regimens	Worse diabetic retinopathy	0.38	0.13	6 years	4
		Nephropathy	0.30	0.10		5
Acute myocardial infarction‡	Streptokinase and Aspirin	Death at 5 weeks	0.134	0.081	5 weeks	19
		Death at 2 years	0.216	0.174	2 years	24
Diastolic blood pressure 115–129 mm Hg§	Antihypertensive drugs	Death, stroke or myocardial infarction	0.1286	0.0137	1.5 years	3
Diastolic blood pressure 90–109 mm Hg¶	Antihypertensive drugs	Death, stroke or myocardial infarction	0.0545	0.0467	5.5 years	128
Independent elderly people**	Comprehensive geriatric home assessment	Long-term nursing home admission	0.10	0.04	3 years	17
Pregnant women with eclampsia††	iv $MgSO_4$ (vs. diazepam)	Recurrent convulsion	0.279	0.132	hours	7
Healthy women ages 50-69‡‡	Breast examination plus mammography	Death from breast cancer	0.00345	0.00252	9 years	1075
Symptomatic high-grade carotid artery stenosis§§	Carotid endarterectomy	Major stroke or death	0.181	0.08	2 years	10
Preterm babies¶¶	Antenatal corticosteroids	Respiratory distress syndrome	0.23	0.13	days	11

To find more examples, and to nominate additions to the databank of NNTs, refer to this textbook's Web Page at: http://cebm.jr2.ox.ac.uk/

* Ann Intern Med 1995;122:561–8; EBM 1995;1:9.
† Diabetes Res Clin Pract 1995;28:103–17
‡ Lancet 1988;2:349–60.
§ JAMA 1967;202:116–22
¶ BMJ 1985;291:97–104.
** N Engl J Med 1995;333:1184–9; EBM 1996;1:87.
†† Lancet 1995;345:1455–63; EBM 1996;1:44.
‡‡ Lancet 1993;341:973–8.
§§ N Engl J Med 1991;325:445–53.
¶¶ Am J Obstet Gynecol 1995;173:322–35; EBM 1996;1:92.

to save one life, about 100 men with no evidence of coronary heart disease for 5 years with aspirin to prevent one heart attack and about 10 patients with symptomatic moderate to severe carotid artery stenosis with endarterectomy to prevent one major or fatal stroke over the following 2 years.

We think that the 'number needed to be treated' (NNT) to prevent one event is the most useful measure of the clinical effort we and our patients must expend in order to help them avoid bad outcomes to their illnesses. Note, however, that this is a measure with real meaning for clinicians, but not for individual patients (who are interested in Ns of 1, not NNTs). Furthermore, because we are focusing here on the magnitude of the treatment effect, rather than on the probability that we have drawn a false-positive conclusion that the treatment is at all effective (when it is not), we should employ confidence intervals around the NNT, specifying the 'limits' within which we can confidently state the true NNT lies (95% of the time), rather than focus just on p-values. Readers who want to brush up on confidence intervals can refer to the Appendix.

Since we are interested in the risks as well as the benefits of treatments, we can generate a parallel 'number needed to harm' or NNH to express the downside of therapy. For example, if anticoagulation carries an annual risk of major bleeding of 2%, the NNH is 1/2% = 50.

Overviews and metaanalyses often provide NNTs, but sometimes only report odds ratios. The latter are not the same as RRRs and can be converted into RRRs only when you know the patient's expected event rate (PEER) by using the formula:

$$NNT = \frac{1 - [PEER \times (1 - OR)]}{(1 - PEER) \times PEER \times (1 - OR)}$$

To help you 'translate' odds ratios to NNTs (without having to crank through this formula), we've summarized several of them in Table 3b3.3.

The NNT from the published report, in light of your own clinical expertise and compared with those in Table 3b3.2, will give you an idea of whether the treatment is potentially

Table 3b3.3 Translating odds ratios to NNTs

		Odds ratio				
		0.9	0.8	0.7	0.6	0.5
Patient's expected event rate (PEER)	.05	209*	104	69	52	41†
	.10	110	54	36	27	21
	.20	61	30	20	14	11
	.30	46	22	14	10	8
	.40	40	19	12	9	7
	.50	38	18	11	8	6
	.70	44	20	13	9	6
	.90	101‡	46	27	18	12§

The numbers in the body of the table are the NNTs for the corresponding odds ratios at that particular patient's expected event rate (PEER).
* The relative risk reduction (RRR) here is 10%.
† The RRR here is 49%.
‡ The RRR here is 1%.
§ The RRR here is 9%.

useful for your patient. In the next chapter, we will show you a very simple way to find out whether this potential is met for your individual patient.

Section 3b4

Is this evidence about harm important?

The main measure that indicates whether valid evidence that a treatment harms some patients is also impressive (and potentially useful clinically) is the strength of the association between receiving the treatment and suffering the adverse effect. Strength here means the risk or odds of the adverse effect with, as opposed to without, exposure to the treatment; the higher the risk or odds, the greater the strength and the more you should be impressed with it.

Different tactics for estimating the strength of association are used in different types of studies and these are shown in Table 3b4.1. In the randomized trial and cohort study, patients who were and were not exposed to the treatment are carefully followed up to find out whether they develop the adverse outcome, with the risk in the treated patients, rela-

Table 3b4.1 Different ways of calculating the strength of an association between a treatment and subsequent adverse outcomes

		Adverse outcome		Totals
		Present (Case)	Absent (Control)	
Exposed to the treatment	Yes (Cohort)	a	b	a+b
	No (Cohort)	c	d	c+d
	Totals	a+c	b+d	a+b+c+d

In a randomized trial or cohort study: relative risk = RR = **[a/(a+b)]/[c/(c+d)]**
In a case-control study: relative odds = RO = **ad/bc**

tive to untreated patients, calculated as **[a/(a+b)]/[c/(c+d)]**. Thus, if 1000 patients receive a treatment and 20 of them have an adverse outcome, **a**=20 and **a/(a+b)** = 20/1000 = 2%; and if just two of 1000 patients with the same condition but receiving a different treatment suffered this adverse outcome, **c**=2 and **c/(c+d)** = 2/1000 = 0.2% and the relative risk = 2%/0.2% or 10. That is, patients receiving the suspect treatment were 10 times as likely to suffer the adverse outcome as patients treated some other way.

In a case-control study, where patients with and without the adverse outcome are selected and tracked backward to their prior treatments, strength (which in this case is called the odds ratio) can only be indirectly estimated as **ad/bc**. For example, if 100 cases of the adverse outcome are assembled and it is discovered that 90 of them had received the suspect treatment, **a**=90 and **c**=10; if 100 control patients, free of the adverse outcome, are also assembled and it is discovered that only 45 of them received the suspect treatment, **b**=45 and **d**=55, and the relative odds = **ad/bc** = (90×55)/(45×10) = 11. That is, patients receiving the suspect treatment are 11 times as likely to suffer the adverse event as patients treated some other way.

How big should relative risks and relative odds become before you should be impressed with them? This question has two answers. First, you'd like to be confident that the relative risk (RR) or relative odds (RO) is really greater than 1 (when RR or RO = 1, the adverse outcome is no greater with than without exposure to the suspect treatment). So, as before, you'd want to be sure that the entire confidence interval remains within a clinically important range of RR or RO. Second, the size of the 'impressive' RR or RO depends on the type of study from which it is generated. Because of the biases we described in case-control studies, you'd want to be sure that the RO was greater than that which could arise from bias alone and you might not want to become impressed with their ROs until they reach 4 or more (some of our colleagues would relax these guides for a serious adverse effect and set them even higher for a trivial one). Since cohort studies are less subject to bias, you might be impressed with RRs of 3 or more in them. And because randomized trials are relatively free of bias, any RR whose confidence interval excludes 1 is impressive and warrants further consideration.

Having decided that you are impressed with both the validity and the strength of the relationship between the suspect treatment and the adverse outcome, you then need to translate this into some measure of the impact of changing your treatment strategy on the occurrence of the adverse outcome and decide whether it is worth the effort required to achieve it. The measures we've employed up to now, the RR and OR, don't provide this information very well and you need to return to the concept of the NNT. In this case you are concerned about a bad outcome and you might want to revise the term to the 'number of patients needed to be treated to produce one episode of harm' or NNH. Our reason for doing this is that the RR and OR are fine for determining whether the link to harm was true, but don't tell us whether the link was clinically important. For example, a cohort study showed that NSAIDS can cause gastrointestinal bleeding and the confidence interval on the relative risk for this adverse outcome included 2. A randomized trial showed that the antiarrhythmic drugs encainide and flecainide can cause death and the confidence interval on the relative risk for this adverse outcome also included 2. But the absolute increase in the risk of bleeding in the former study was small, at about 0.05%, which translates to an NNH of 2000 to cause one more GI bleed, whereas the absolute increase in the risk of death in the latter trial was 4.7% or an NNH of 21 to cause one additional death! Clearly, similar RRs or ORs can lead to very different NNHs and you need the latter as well as the former to make your clinical decision about your patient.

That final step of integrating this external evidence with your clinical expertise is discussed in Section 4.4.

Further reading

Levine M, Walter S D, Lee H, Haines T, Holbrook A, Moyer V for the Evidence-Based Medicine Working Group. Users' guides to the medical literature: IV. How to use an article about harm. JAMA 1994; 271: 1615–19.

Section 4.1

Can you apply this valid, important evidence about a diagnostic test in caring for your patient?

Having found a valid systematic review or individual report about a diagnostic test and decided that its accuracy is sufficiently high to be useful, how do you integrate it with your individual clinical expertise and apply it to your patient?

There are three questions whose answers dictate this determination, summarized in Table 4.1.1. First, is the diagnostic test available, affordable, accurate and precise in your setting? You obviously can't order a test that's not available but even if it is, you may want to check around to be sure that it's performed and interpreted in a competent, reproducible fashion and that its potential consequences (see below) justify its cost. Moreover, diagnostic tests often behave differently among different subsets of patients, generating higher likelihood ratios in later stages of florid disease and lower likelihood ratios in early, mild stages. This is another reason why multilevel likelihood ratios are helpful, as there are at least theoretical reasons why they should suffer less distortion from this cause. Finally, it is known that at least some diagnostic tests based on symptoms or signs lose power as patients move from primary care to secondary and tertiary care. Reference back to Table 3b1.1 can show you why: if patients are referred onward in part because of symptoms, their primary care clinicians will be sending along patients in both cells **a** and **b** and subsequent evaluations of the accuracy of their symptoms will tend to show falling specificity due to the referral of patients with false-positive findings. If you think that any of these factors may be operating, you can try out what you judge to be clinically sensible variations in the likelihood ratios for your test result and see whether the results alter your post-test probabilities in a way that changes your diagnosis (the short-hand term for this sort of exploration is 'sensitivity analysis').

Table 4.1.1 Questions to answer in applying a valid diagnostic test to an individual patient

1. **Is the diagnostic test available, affordable, accurate and precise in your setting?**
2. **Can you generate a clinically sensible estimate of your patient's pretest probability:**
   - **from practice data?**
   - **from personal experience?**
   - **from the report itself?**
   - **from clinical speculation?**
3. **Will the resulting post-test probabilities affect your management and help your patient?**
   - **Could it move you across a test–treatment threshold?**
   - **Would your patient be a willing partner in carrying it out?**
   - **Would the consequences of the test help your patient reach their goals in all this?**

The second question you need to answer is whether you can generate a clinically sensible estimate of your patient's pretest probability. Sometimes you've actually got the data on pretest probabilities from your practice or institution. That's wonderful when it exists and constitutes a reason to consider keeping some records on the pretest probabilities for important diagnoses you eventually make for the specific presenting complaints in which you'd consider this sort of diagnostic test. Sometimes, you've had enough experience both to be able to make this estimation based on your own experience and to know how your estimate can be distorted by your last case (either way, depending on whether you ruled in or ruled out the diagnosis), your most dramatic or embarrassing case (usually this either distorts your pretest odds upwards or makes you reluctant to quit testing until the post-test odds are vanishingly small) or by whether you are an expert in the evaluation or care of patients with this diagnosis (which usually makes you reluctant to miss one).

Early in your career or when you haven't previously encountered this diagnostic situation, you'll be less certain about your patient's pretest probability. When that hap pens, you can try one or more of the following. First, if your setting and patient closely resemble those that appeared in the report, you can use its pretest probability. Or if your patient is a bit different from those in the study, you can use its pretest probability as a starting point and again set off on a sensitivity analysis using clinically sensible variations in pretest probabilities and determining their impact on the test's usefulness. As before, the issue here is not whether your patient is exactly like those in the report, but whether they are so different that the report is of no help in making the diagnosis. Finally, you may simply go straight to a sensitivity analysis in which you plug the likelihood ratios from your report into a range of sensible pretest probabilities and see what the likely range of post-test probabilities will be (perhaps using the entries in Table 3b1.4 on page 124 to help you).

The final question you need to answer is: Will the resulting post-test probabilities affect your management and help your patient? The elements of this answer are three. First, could its results move you across some threshold that would cause you to stop all further testing? Two thresholds should be borne in mind. If the diagnostic test was negative or generated a likelihood ratio well below 1.0, the post-test probability might become so low that you would abandon the diagnosis it was pursuing and turn to other diagnostic possibilities. Put in terms of thresholds, this negative test result has moved you from above to below the 'test threshold' and you won't do any more tests for that diagnostic possibility. On the other hand, if the diagnostic test came back positive or generated a high likelihood ratio, the post-test probability might become so high that you would also abandon further testing because you'd made your diagnosis and would now move to choosing the most appropriate therapy; in these terms, you've now crossed from below to above the 'treatment threshold'. It's only if your diagnostic test result leaves you stranded between the test and treatment thresholds that you'd continue to pursue that initial diagnosis by performing other tests. Although there are some very fancy ways of calculating test and treatment thresholds from test accuracy and the risks and benefits of correct and incorrect

diagnostic conclusions,* intuitive test–treatment thresholds are commonly used by experienced clinicians and are another example of individual clinical expertise.

You may not cross a test–treatment threshold until you've performed several different diagnostic tests and here is where another nice property of the likelihood ratio comes into play. Because the post-test odds for the first diagnostic test you apply are the pretest odds for your second diagnostic test, you needn't switch back and forth between odds and probabilities between tests. You can simply keep multiplying the running product by the likelihood ratio generated from the next test. For example, when a 45-year-old man walks into your office his pretest probability of ≥75% stenosis of one or more of his coronary arteries is about 6%. Suppose that he gives you a history of atypical chest pain (only two of the three symptoms of substernal chest discomfort, brought on by exertion, and relieved in <10 minutes by rest: a likelihood ratio of about 13) and that his exercise ECG reveals 2.2 mm of non-sloping ST-segment depression (a likelihood ratio of about 11). Then his post-test probability for coronary stenosis is his pretest probability [converted into odds] times the product of the likelihood ratios generated from his history (13) and exercise ECG (11), with the resulting post-test odds converted back to probabilities (through dividing by its value + 1): $(0.06 / 0.94) \times 13 \times 11 = 9.13 / 10.13 = 90\%$. The final result of these calculations is strictly accurate as long as the diagnostic tests being combined are 'independent' (that is, the probability of a specific result on the second is the same for any result on the first) and we know intuitively that this is not true for most of the diagnostic tests we apply in sequences aiming toward a single diagnosis. Accordingly, we'd want the calculated post-test probability at the end of this sequence to be comfortably above our treatment threshold before we would act upon it. This additional example of how likelihood ratios make lots of implicit diagnostic reasoning explicit is another argument in favor of generating overall

* See the recommendations for further reading or N Engl J Med 1980; 302: 1109.

likelihood ratios for sequences or clusters of diagnostic tests, as suggested back in Section 3b1.

We hope that you involved your patient as you worked your way through all the foregoing considerations that lead you to think that the diagnostic test is worth considering. If you haven't, you certainly need to do so now. Every diagnostic test involves some invasion of privacy and some are embarrassing, painful or dangerous. You'll have to be sure that the patient is an informed, willing partner in the undertaking.

Finally, the ultimate question to ask about using any diagnostic test is whether its consequences (reassurance when negative, labeling and possibly generating awful diagnostic and prognostic news if positive, leading to further diagnostic tests and treatments, etc.) will help your patient achieve their goals of therapy. Included here are considerations of how subsequent interventions match clinical guidelines or restrictions on access to therapy designed to optimize the use of finite resources for all members of your society.

Further reading

Jaeschke R, Guyatt G H, Sackett D L for the Evidence-Based Medicine Working Group. Users' guides to the medical literature. VI. How to use an article about a diagnostic test. B. What are the results and will they help me in caring for my patients? JAMA 1994; 271: 703–7.

Section 4.2

Can you apply this valid, important evidence about prognosis in caring for your patient?

Having decided that the evidence you tracked down about prognosis is both valid and important, you now can consider how to use it in your clinical practice. Two guides can help you make these judgments; they appear in Table 4.2.1 and will be considered here.

First, were the study patients sufficiently similar to your own? The first guide asks you to compare your patients to those in the article and since presumably you know your patients well, this means trying to get to know the study patients well enough to compare them. Look for descriptions of the study sample, including the patients' demographics and important clinical characteristics. The more the study patients are like your patients, the more readily you can apply the results to your patients. Inevitably, some differences will turn up, so how similar is similar enough? To help you with this judgment, as in other places in this book, we suggest that you try this question framed the other way: are the study patients so different from yours that you'd expect their outcomes to be so different that they wouldn't be any use to you in making prognostic predictions about your patients?

Second, will this evidence make a clinically important impact on your conclusions about what to offer or tell your patient? If the evidence suggests a good prognosis when patients (especially in the early stages of disease) remain untreated, that could strongly influence your discussion of treatment options with them. If, on the other hand, prognostic information derived from a control group in a randomized trial suggests a gloomy prognosis when no definitive therapy is instituted, your message to your patient would reflect this fact. And even when the prognostic evidence doesn't lead to a treat/don't treat decision, valid evidence is always useful in providing your patient or their family with the information they want to have about what the future is likely to hold for them and their illness.

Table 4.2.1 Can you apply this valid, important evidence about prognosis in caring for your patient?

1. **Were the study patients similar to your own?**
2. **Will this evidence make a clinically important impact on your conclusions about what to offer or tell your patient?**

Further reading

Laupacis A, Wells G, Richardson W S, Tugwell P for the Evidence-Based Medicine Working Group. Users' guides to the medical literature. V. How to use an article about prognosis. JAMA 1994; 272: 234–7.

Section 4.3

Can you apply this valid, important evidence about a treatment in caring for your patient?

In deciding whether valid, potentially useful results apply to your patient, you need once again to integrate the evidence with your clinical expertise. As shown in Table 4.3.1, there are two elements to this integration. The first estimates the impact of the treatment on patients just like yours and the second compares the values and preferences of your patient with the regimen and its consequences.

Estimating the impact of a valid, important treatment result on an individual patient

This element poses two additional questions: Do these results apply to your patient? How great would the potential benefit of therapy actually be for your individual patient?

Do these results apply to your patient?

Your patient wasn't in the trial that established the efficacy of this treatment. Maybe (because of their age, sex, comorbidity, disease severity or for a host of other sociodemographic, biologic or clinical reasons) they wouldn't even have been eligible for the trial. How can you extrapolate* from the external evidence to your individual patient? Rather than slavishly asking: 'Would my patient satisfy the eligibility criteria for the trial?' and rejecting its usefulness if they didn't exactly fit every one of them, we'd suggest bringing in some of your knowledge of human biology and

* Some teachers call this 'generalizing' from the trial, but really it's 'particularizing' to an individual patient, not generalizing to all patients, everywhere. Accordingly, we'll use the more generic term 'extrapolating'.

Table 4.3.1 Are these valid, potentially useful results applicable to your patient?

1. **Do these results apply to your patient?**
   - **Is your patient so different from those in the trial that its results can't help you?**
   - **How great would the potential benefit of therapy actually be for your individual patient?**
2. **Are your patient's values and preferences satisfied by the regimen and its consequences?**
   - **Do your patient and you have a clear assessment of their values and preferences?**
   - **Are they met by this regimen and its consequences?**

clinical experience, turning the question around and asking: 'Is my patient so different from those in the trial that its results cannot help me make my treatment decision?' Pharmacogenetics aside, there are very few situations in which you would expect a drug or diet or operation to produce qualitatively different results in patients inside a trial and those who don't quite fit its eligibility criteria. Only if you conclude that your patient is so different from those in the study that its results simply don't inform your treatment decision should you discard its results.

What about subgroups?

Sometimes treatments appear to benefit some subgroups of patients but not others. For example, some of the early trials of aspirin for transient ischemic attacks suggested that this drug was efficacious in men but not in women. As is usually the case, this 'qualitative' difference in the effects of therapy (helpful for one group but useless or harmful in another) was a chance finding and later trials and overviews confirmed that aspirin is efficacious in women. The results from megatrials and overviews suggest that extrapolations from the overall results of individual trials usually are correct when applied to subgroups of patients in those trials. If you think that you may be dealing with one of the exceptions to this rule and that the treatment you're examining really does work in a qualitatively different way among

Table 4.3.2 Should you believe apparent qualitative differences in the efficacy of therapy in some subgroups of patients?

Only if you can say 'yes' to all of the following:
1. **Does it really make biologic and clinical sense?**
2. **Is the qualitative difference both clinically (beneficial for some but useless or harmful for others) and statistically significant?**
3. **Was it hypothesized before the study began (rather than the product of dredging the data) and has it been confirmed in other, independent studies?**
4. **Was it one of just a few subgroup analyses carried out in this study?**

different patients, you should apply the guides in Table 4.3.2. In particular, unless this difference in response makes biologic sense, was hypothesized before the trial and has been confirmed in a second, independent trial, we'd suggest that you accept the treatment's overall efficacy as the best estimate of its efficacy in your patient.

So, unless there is some really powerful biologic reason for you to think that the treatment, if accepted by your patient, would be totally ineffectual or act in the opposing direction from the way it acted in patients in the study, we think you have good grounds for extrapolating the *direction* of the effect of the treatment on your patient's illness. Having decided that the direction of the treatment effect is likely to be the same as that observed in the study, you can now turn to considering whether that effect is likely to be great or small.

How great would the potential benefit of therapy be for your individual patient?

The trial report informed you about how the treatment worked in the average patient in the trial. How can you translate this to the probable treatment effect in your individual patient? We suggest that the measure we used to decide whether the treatment was potentially useful, the number of patients you need to treat (NNT) to prevent one bad outcome, is useful here. The trick is to translate the NNT

from the study into an NNT that fits your patient. You can do this the longer, harder (and maybe more accurate*) way or the quick and easy (but maybe less accurate) way.

The long way is to estimate the absolute susceptibility of your individual patient for developing the bad outcome over a period of time equal to the duration of the study. If the study you're using had a placebo or no-treatment group or subgroup with features like your patient, you could use their susceptibility† for this purpose. Another way would be to carry out a literature search to find a paper on the prognosis of patients like yours and use that figure. Either way, you'd take the resulting susceptibility (you could express it as a decimal fraction or a percentage, whichever you're more comfortable using) and multiply it by the RRR from the study. The result is the ARR and you can invert it to get the NNT. For example, if you find a prognosis paper suggesting that the susceptibility of your patient for a bad outcome is about 0.4 (the term we use to describe that susceptibility is the 'patient expected event rate' or PEER, so PEER = 40%) over a period of time equal to the duration of the trial that generated an RRR of 50%. Assuming that this RRR applies regardless of the susceptibility of patients in that trial, the ARR is PEER × RRR = 40% × 50% = 20% and the corresponding NNT is 1/ARR = 1/20% = 5 and you'd need to treat just five patients like yours for that length of time to prevent one event. If you would like to avoid these calculations, you can use the nomogram that appears in Figure 4.3.1. But there is an even easier way to estimate an NNT for patients like yours.

As we stated in the previous chapter, one of the reasons why the NNT is useful when interpreting the results of treatment trials is the ease with which it can be extrapolated to your own practice and to individual patients outside the trials. Through some very simple arithmetic, you can estimate NNTs for specific patients. All you need do is estimate the

* We're not being cute here. We all are pretty new at this and really don't know!

† Some people, especially when they use a control group to estimate susceptibility, call it 'baseline risk'.

susceptibility of your individual patient (if they were to receive just the control treatment) relative to the average control patient in the reported trial and convert this estimate into a decimal fraction we'll call F (if you judge your patient to be twice as susceptible as those in the trial, F = 2; if your patient is only half as susceptible as the average control patient in the trial, F = 0.5, and if just like the patients in the trial, F = 1). As long as the treatment produces a constant relative risk reduction across the spectrum of susceptibilities,* the NNT for your patient is simply the reported NNT divided by F. Going back to our intensive insulin example in Section 3b3, we learned that a group of clinical investigators had to treat 15 diabetics with intensive insulin regimens for 6.5 years in order to prevent one of them from developing diabetic neuropathy (NNT=15). If you judge that your patient was only half as susceptible as patients in that trial, F = 0.5 and NNT/F = 15/0.5 = 30, so 30 of these less susceptible patients would need to be treated for about 6.5 years with the intensive insulin regimen to prevent one of them from going on to develop neuropathy.

Comparing the values and preferences of your patient with the regimen and its consequences

A return to Table 4.3.1 identifies the steps to be taken here. You and your patient need to achieve a clear assessment of their values and preferences and then determine whether they will be served by the regimen in question. Sometimes the answer will be evident in a few seconds: for a patient having a heart attack, the value of survival and the preference for a simple, low-risk intervention like aspirin, given the efficacy of this regimen, usually makes this decision quickly agreed and acted upon. Other times the answer will take weeks and several visits to sort out: radiation or

* This is a big assumption and we're only beginning to learn when assuming a constant RRR is appropriate (for lots of medical treatments like antihypertensive drugs) and inappropriate (for some operations like carotid endarterectomy, where the RRR rises with increasing susceptibility).

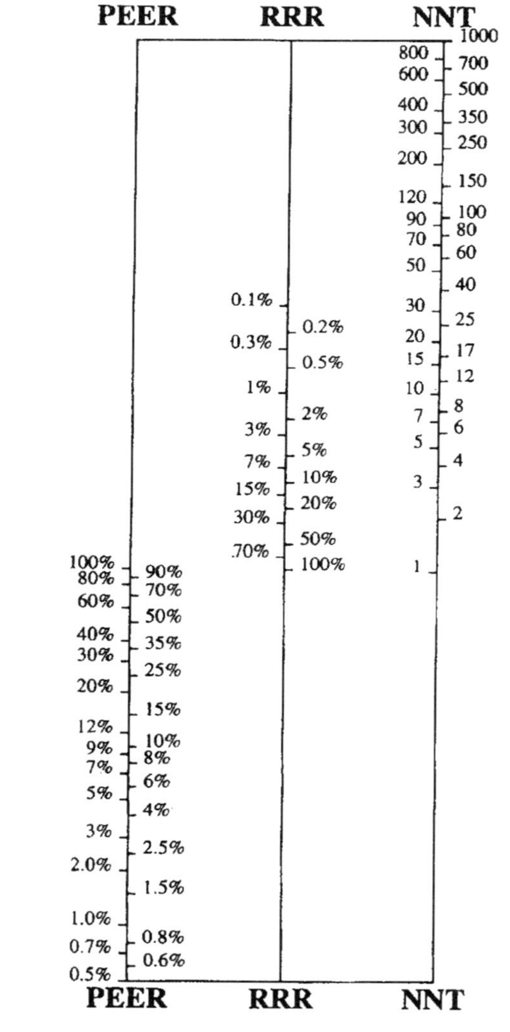

Figure 4.3.1 A nomogram for determining NNTs. Reprinted with permission from Chatellier G et al. The number needed to treat: a clinically useful nomogram in its proper context. BMJ 1996; 312: 426–9.

adjuvant chemotherapy for stage II carcinoma of the breast or transurethral resection of the prostate for moderate symptoms of prostatism.

Section 4.4

Can you apply this valid, important evidence about harm in caring for your patient?

In deciding whether and how to apply valid, potentially important results of a critical appraisal about a harmful treatment to an individual patient, four aspects of individual clinical expertise are important and they are listed in Table 4.4.1.

First, you need to decide whether the results of your critical appraisal can be extrapolated to your patient. As before, the issue is not whether your patient would have met all the inclusion criteria for the systematic review or individual study that demonstrated the harmful effect of the treatment, but whether your patient is so different from those in the report that its results provide no useful guidance for you.

Second, you need to estimate your patient's risk of the adverse outcome relative to the patients in the report. As we described in Section 4.3, if you can express this as a decimal fraction we'll call F (if your patient is twice the risk of those in the report, F=2; if half the risk, F=0.5; if the same risk, F=1) you can then simply divide the number of patients needed to be treated to produce one episode of harm (NNH) from the report by F. If, for example, you decided that a patient you're considering placing on an NSAID is at four times the risk of an upper GI bleed as those in a cohort study

Table 4.4.1 Should these valid, potentially important results of a critical appraisal about a harmful drug change the treatment of an individual patient?

1. **Can the study results be extrapolated to this patient?**
2. **What are this patient's risks of the adverse outcome?**
3. **What are this patient's preferences, concerns and expectations from this treatment?**
4. **What alternative treatments are available?**

that generated an NNH of 2000, the appropriate NNH for your patient becomes 2000/4 = 500.

Third, as with all clinical decisions, you need to identify and incorporate your patient's preferences, concerns and expectations into your recommendation. If they are 'risk-averse', on the one hand, or willing to gamble side-effects to gain possible treatment benefit, on the other, your discussions of the risks and benefits of the same treatment, even among patients with identical NNHs, may lead to very different treatment plans. At this point you can further modify NNH (or its F, whichever you are more comfortable dealing with) to take into account both your own and your patient's thoughts about the comparative health impacts of the treatment's adverse effect and the clinical event it was being used to prevent in the first place (represented by its NNT). If your patient is risk averse or if either of you thinks that the treatment's adverse effect (e.g. an intracranial bleed from anticoagulants) is 2–3 times as severe as the event the treatment was intended to prevent (recurrent deep vein thrombosis), you could double or triple the F for the NNH (or cut the NNH by 1/2 or 2/3) and then see how it compares with the NNT. If, on the other hand, your patient is a risk taker or the adverse treatment effect (e.g. cough from an ACE inhibitor) was only 1% as severe as the event the treatment was intended to prevent (death from heart failure), you could reduce the F for the NNH to 0.01 or multiply the NNH by 100.* In either case, the comparison of the treatment's 'adjusted' NNH with its NNT becomes very informative. If a treatment's NNH, after all this adjustment, is lower than its NNT, shouldn't you be considering some therapeutic alternatives? If your time and resources permit, this would be an ideal situation in which to carry out a clinical decision analysis.

Even if the adjusted NNH exceeds the NNT, you still ought to identify the possible alternative treatments (including no treatment!) you could offer your patient instead of the one

* In similar fashion, when a treatment (e.g. NSAIDs for arthritis) causes multiple adverse effects, you would apply a smaller F (or higher NNH) for a minor one (e.g. indigestion) than a major one (e.g. GI hemorrhage).

that produces this adverse effect. If a patient experienced wheezing when their hypertension was treated with a beta-blocker, it is easy to substitute another antihypertensive drug that is free of this side-effect. On the other hand, the alternatives to oral contraceptives for temporary conception control may not be acceptable to your patient, despite the small but real risk of thromboembolism from these drugs.

Further reading

Levine M, Walter S D, Lee H, Haines T, Holbrook A, Moyer V for the Evidence-Based Medicine Working Group. Users' guides to the medical literature. IV. How to use an article about harm. JAMA 1994; 271: 1615–19.

Section 4.6

Teaching methods relevant to the clinical application of the results of critical appraisals to individual patients

In this section we will present some strategies and tactics for teaching learners how to apply the results of their critical appraisals to patients. Because EBM begins and ends with patients, it is natural for us to use patient encounters for closing this loop. The message here is that critical appraisal and other elements of EBM are integral components of the everyday bedside and other clinical discussions of how to diagnose and manage patients and not peripheral topics to be discussed at other places and only when time permits. We will start with some obvious clinical situations, but then move progressively farther afield to demonstrate that closely similar strategies and tactics can be applied to a wide variety of teaching and learning situations. Finally, we will describe how several centers and academic consortia around the world operate 5-day workshops on how to practice EBM.

Working rounds on individual patients

First we will consider the 'working round' in which a clinical team review the problems and progress of patients on a clinical service or in an outpatient setting. These are held in various formats. On an inpatient unit, they might consist of a walking round in which every patient on the service is briefly presented, seen and discussed. In an outpatient setting, they might focus on a single patient who has been asked to stay behind or might consider the entire session's patients after they've left. Finally, they might be quite informal gatherings over coffee in which discussions around patients are tagged onto meetings that deal largely with administrative and housekeeping tasks. When the available time is in harmony with the numbers of patients to be seen

(or at least discussed), these can provide excellent opportunities for teaching and learning EBM. Often, however, time is short and the list of patients long and in those circumstances many services adopt a two-stage approach in which they begin by sitting down and quickly reviewing the patient list and then focus on just those patients in whom major decisions have to be made. In either format, patients are presented (and, if available, examined), followed by discussions in which management decisions are taken and defended with the best available evidence. How might these discussions be organized to maximize the opportunities for learning and practicing EBM? Two tactics are useful here.

The first ties EBM to the presentation of the patient. Back in Chapter 1 we described how the educational prescription could be used to initiate finding and critically appraising evidence and in Table 1.5 we showed how it could form the final element in presenting a new patient. In a similar fashion, as shown in Table 4.6.1, filling that educational Rx can form the final element of presenting a patient already known to the clinical service. In this fashion, the scientific justification for a diagnostic or therapeutic course of action becomes part of describing the past and planning the future care of the patient and serves the decision-making as well as educational requirements of the meeting.

The second tactic concerns the actual presentation of the evidence. The busier the service, the more important that evidence central to management decisions is concisely and quickly presented. This is where the CATs (introduced back in Section 3b7) can come in so handy.* After hearing about and (if possible) examining the patient, the team can gather around the resulting CAT, quickly decide whether its clinical bottom line applies, make the management decision and get on to the next patient (requesting copies of CATs for further study or later use).

* For greatest effect, CATs have to be produced in real time while decisions are being made (often easier between visits in ambulatory settings than overnight in inpatient settings). To speed their production, a CAT-Maker is available on disk or via the Website at the Oxford Centre for Evidence-Based Medicine (http://cebm.jr2.ox.ac.uk/).

Table 4.6.1 A guide for learners in presenting an 'OLD'* patient at follow-up rounds

The presentation should summarize 20 things in less than 2 minutes:

1. **The patient's surname.**
2. **Their age.**
3. **Their gender.**
4. **Their occupation/social role.**
5. **When they were admitted.**
6. **Their chief complaint(s) that led directly to their admission.**
7. **The number of ACTIVE PROBLEMS that they have at the present time.**
   And then, for each ACTIVE PROBLEM (a problem could be a symptom, sign, event, diagnosis, injury, psychological state, social predicament, etc.):
8. **Its most important symptoms, if any.**
9. **Its most important signs, if any.**
10. **The results of diagnostic or other exploratory/confirmatory investigations.**
11. **The explanation (diagnosis or state) for the problem.**
12. **The treatment plan instituted for the problem.**
13. **The response to this treatment plan.**
14. **The future plans for managing this problem.**
    Repeat 8–14 for each ACTIVE PROBLEM.
15. **Your plans for discharge, posthospital care and follow-up.**
16. **Whether you've filled the educational prescription that you requested when this patient was admitted (in order to better understand the patient's pathophysiology, clinical findings, diagnosis, prognosis, therapy, prevention of recurrence, quality of care or other important issue in order to become a better clinician).**
    If so:
17. **How you found the relevant evidence.**
18. **What you found. The clinical bottom line derived from that evidence.**
19. **Your critical appraisal of that evidence for its VALIDITY and APPLICABILITY.**
20. **How that critically appraised evidence will alter your care of that (or the next similar) patient.**
    If not, when you are going to fill it.

* That is, a patient already known to the service.

The sorts of words you might use:

A. Mr/Mrs/Ms/Prof/PC 11111 is a 22222 year-old 33333 44444 who was admitted on 55555 with the chief complaint of 66666.

B. They have 77777 Active Problems.

C. The first active problem is ________________.
It is characterized by 88888 and 99999 and we performed a __________ which revealed 10–10–10–10. We decided that the cause for this problem was 11–11–11–11 and we started 12–12–12–12, to which he/she responded with 13–13–13–13. We plan to 14–14–14–14.

D. The second/third/fourth active problem is __________ (repeat 8–14)

E. At the time of her/his admission, I didn't understand ______________ as well as I'd like to and I requested an educational Rx to answer the question:
____
I found the relevant evidence by 17–17–17–17 and its clinical bottom line is 18–18–18–18. I believe that this bottom line is/is not valid because 19a–19a–19a–19a and I believe that it is/is not applicable because 19b–19b–19b–19b. I therefore plan to manage this and future, similar patients by 20–20–20–20.

Small groups and 'academic half-days'

Quite often, learners from different clinical teams gather at regularly scheduled educational sessions to receive general instruction in the evaluation and management of patients. The numbers of learners at these sessions can range from a handfull to a hall-full and running them on a 'set-piece' lecture format can tax the ability of the teachers to stay enthused and the ability of the learners to stay awake. An alternative approach builds on the self-directed, problem-based EBM learning orientation and runs as follows:

1. Learners are asked to identify clinical problems for which they are uncertain about the best way to diagnose or manage affected patients (stating their uncertainties in the form of clinical questions, as in Chapter 1, specifying the patient, the intervention and the outcome of interest to them). Training programs employing this approach report a distinct

pattern in the problems that learners identify. Early on, postgraduates identify medical emergencies in which they are unsure of their skills at diagnosing and managing life-threatening situations. Many programs anticipate these concerns and have basic and advanced cardiac and/or trauma support training at the ready.

2. Once the foregoing concerns are addressed, postgraduates identify a wide array of management problems in which they are not sure how to treat patients with specific disorders, followed by clinical problems in diagnosis, prognosis and etiology (especially for iatrogenic disorders). Occasionally, interest is expressed in a locally occurring quality of care study or audit, in their own continuing education, and in health economics. When several learners identify the same clinical situation,* it joins the schedule for a future session and the following processes occur:

- Acting in rotation, one or more of the learners takes on the task of searching the clinical literature for valid, relevant systematic reviews or primary articles on the clinical problem. Along the way, with help from librarians as needed, they develop and hone their skills in searching for the best evidence.
- With faculty guidance, they pick the one or two articles of highest validity and relevance and these, along with a description of the clinical problem, are copied and distributed to everyone to be studied in advance of the session.
- At that session, and again with faculty guidance as needed, they lead the discussion of the validity and potential usefulness of the evidence presented in the paper. Presenters often aid the discussion by introducing CATs or other summaries and displays of the most relevant evidence. This critical appraisal is integrated with discussions of the related pathophysiology and clinical skills, with the final objective of generating a common, evidence-based approach to the clinical

* Part of an initial session can be devoted to reaching consensus on priority clinical problems and such discussions can be repeated as current topics are exhausted and new topics arise.

problem. In some cases, the learners may want to work with senior clinicians to generate and circulate their own guidelines for future use.

Over the years, teachers of EBM have discovered lots of ways *not* to teach effectively and several ways that seem to work. We have summarized them in the form of a set of teaching tips, which appear in Table 4.6.2.

Journal clubs

Journal clubs are dying or dead in many clinical centers, especially when they rely on a rota through which members are asked to summarize the latest issues of preassigned journals. When you think about it, that sort of journal club is run by the postman, not the clinicians or patients, and it is no wonder that it is becoming extinct. On the other hand, a few journal clubs are flourishing and a growing number of them are designed and conducted along EBM lines. They operate like the 'academic half-days' described above.

Each meeting of the journal club has three parts:

1. In one part, journal club members describe patients who exemplify clinical situations which they are uncertain how best to diagnose or manage. This discussion continues until there is consensus that a particular clinical problem,* which we'll call problem C, is worth the time and effort necessary to find its solution. Then either the member who nominated the problem or another member, based on a rota, takes responsibility for performing a search for the best evidence on problem C.

2. In a second part, the results of the evidence search on last session's problem (we'll call it problem B) are shared in the form of photocopies of the abstracts of 4–6 systematic reviews, original articles or other evidence. Club members decide which one or two pieces of evidence are worth studying and arrangements are made to get copies of the clinical problem statement and best evidence to all members well in advance of the next meeting.

* Stated (as in Chapter 1) in terms of a patient, an intervention (and a comparison intervention if appropriate) and an outcome.

Table 4.6.2 Some teaching tips for EBM*

Motivating learning

A. Keep the session relevant and meaningful to learners.

1. Select (or help them track down) articles that relate to patients in their care and pick 'good' articles. Types of good articles for critical appraisal purposes (in decreasing order of their liveliness potential) include those that provide:
   - ground-breaking but solid evidence at the forefront of clinical practice (especially if not yet in widespread use);
   - solid evidence that a common practice is worthless;
   - solid evidence that a common practice ought to be questioned;
   - for common or controversial practices:
     (i) a pair of articles – a bad one to trash, maybe after reading no further than the methods, plus a good one to use for decision making or,
     (ii) a bad article with high trash titres but nonetheless the best one available;
   - NOTE: solid evidence supporting current practice is an excellent place to start (so as to avoid cynicism or nihilism) but risks boring more experienced learners.
2. Start sessions with a patient's problem (real or simulated) and end sessions by coming to a conclusion about how to manage the patient.
3. Save time for closure. Come to closure about both the article and the patient. Closure does not necessarily require unanimous agreement. The group may agree that the evidence is fairly solid but still not agree on individuals' decisions for the patient in the scenario.
4. If a methodological issue comes up that may sidetrack the discussion, ask the group how they want to handle it (usually it can be deferred and discussed with just the subset of learners who are interested in deeper methodology).

B. Keep the learners active.

1. Ask the learners to vote on what they would do clinically before the article is discussed. Ask them to write down their recommendations and pass in their scripts anonymously to avoid embarrassment.
2. When someone asks a question, NEVER ridicule them.
3. Turn questions back to the person asking or to the entire group: 'What does the group think?', 'Can anyone help out here?'
4. Call on people only when they feel comfortable and know it is 'OK' not to know.
5. Ask challenging (but not intimidating) open-ended questions. 'What do the authors mean by a randomized trial?' vs 'Is this a randomized trial?'
6. When bias might be present in an article, ask the group to decide if it might be important. If present, in what direction would it influence the results, i.e. would it widen or narrow a difference between groups? Do a worst case scenario analysis. Would this bias, if present and affecting all members of a group, reverse the analysis? (In other words, could this bias be a fatal flaw?)
7. When discussing diagnostic tests, go right to likelihood ratios (omit sensitivity, specificity, prevalence, etc.), go straight to the relevant 2×2 table and help the learners generate the appropriate proportions and calculations, asking them as you go along to express what the calculations mean in words. Only afterwards ask them to put names to these concepts, like sensitivity, specificity, etc.*
8. Summarize specific points during the session; check if it's OK to move on to the next topic. Stop from time to time to synthesize and summarize to show the group that there is a set of take-home messages even though full closure may not have occurred.
9. Time out: when particular problems or successes are occurring in the group dynamic, call 'time out' to divert attention to the group process rather than the clinical problem. Examine with the group what is occurring in the interaction, then call 'time in' to return to the clinical problem. Time outs can be especially useful when the teacher senses tension: call a time out, tell the group you sense tension and ask them what's going on.

C. Show your enthusiasm for critical appraisal in general and look for opportunities to compliment your specific set of learners and the work they are doing.

D. Novelty (once your team become adept at critical appraisal).

1. Use more controversial clinical topics and articles.
2. Use articles that come to different conclusions on the same topic.
3. In non-clinical situations, use 'role play' and scenarios. For role play, if people are reluctant, ask them to just play themselves, in the situations they find in their daily work life. Other situations to try include: courtrooms and malpractice claims, formal debates, point-counterpoint (appoint individuals to each role), hostile residents (or consultants!) on teaching rounds.
4. Introduce a 'quick challenge' for 'snap diagnosis': for an article with a fatal flaw, especially if you sense or discover that the group has not prepared in advance, start the session with: 'Quick, is there a fatal flaw in this paper and if so, what is it?'

Learning climate

A. Learners must feel comfortable identifying and addressing their limitations.

1. Be open about your own limitations and the things you don't know.
2. Use educational prescriptions (see page 33).
3. Periodically, make it a point to say that no one knows everything and that is why we are all here.
4. Encourage people to ask questions.
5. Have fun.
6. Provide feedback. Nod your head or make some reinforcing comment, especially when a correct response is given to a question or someone brings up an important issue.

B. Fight 'critical appraisal nihilism' ('No study is perfect, so what good is any of the literature?').

1. Select good articles, especially at the start.
2. Put the article into perspective in terms of what is known in the research area. This may be the first clinical trial of a new treatment.
3. Ask learners what they would look for in (or, if they are keen to do research, how they would design) a better study on this clinical issue.
4. Remind the learners that they have to use what is available in the literature for clinical decision making. Application of critical appraisal to clinical decision making is a positive process; not using critical appraisal can result in mindless adoption of faulty practices. Mindlessness is more nihilistic than questioning and seeking the right answer.
5. Separate innocent and possible problems from fatal flaws.
6. Help learners sort the literature and the clinical practice it supports into three categories: definitely useful, incompletely tested and definitely useless.
7. Remind the learners that it may be the editors' and not the authors' fault that insufficient information is provided in the published article.

---

* Credit for the original compilation of this list goes to Martha Gerrity and Valerie Lawrence.

* Like lots of the elements of EBM, these concepts are not difficult but their jargon can be mystifying, so if you can orient students to the numbers and get them to say what they mean, you can later apply the usual terms, hopefully now demystified.

C. How to handle statistics.

1. Note the difference between statistical significance and clinical importance.
2. Use the 'statistics isn't important' technique. As a tutor, don't permit the session to turn into an attempt to teach statistics. Tell group members that study methods, samples, clinical measurements, follow-up and clinical conclusions are what's important and that statistics are merely tools to help these processes. If good methods were used, the investigators probably went to the effort to use good statistics (the 'trust 'em' mode). If bad methods were used, good statistics could never rescue the study (garbage in/garbage out, the frog is a frog and not a prince).
3. Suggest the quick and dirty sample size calculations such as the inverse rule of 3 on page 107.

Group control of the session

A. Discuss the goals of the session at its beginning and check along the way on whether it's making progress, especially if the discussion seems to be getting off track.

B. Learners' agenda versus teacher's agenda.

1. Try to go with the learners' agenda as much as possible. They will not learn all there is to know about critical appraisal in one session – remember how long it took you to learn it.
2. Let the group generate their own agenda for a specific session. This may lead into uncharted territory but learning will often be increased. The unlikely outcome is that closure may not be achieved, so be on guard to reassure (and, if you can't stand the chaos, provide direction).
3. Evaluate at the end to see if all goals were accomplished and how the next session could be more productive, more learner centered, more active, more stimulating and more fun.

C. When individuals try to dominate the discussion, put down others or 'know it all', take a 'time out' and ask the group to discuss individual responsibilities to the group. This should facilitate discussion of individual responsibilities and provide energy for individuals to take more responsibility (by the loud ones lightening up and the quiet ones contributing more).

D. When individuals or the whole group clam up and won't participate (not unusual at the first session).

1. Wait the 'magic 17 seconds'. No one can stand silence for more than about 5 seconds and the tutor who knows

(and believes!) this can outwait any group or member, no matter how long it takes. Refrain from jumping in to fill the silence yourself or they'll know that they don't have to take responsibility for their learning.
2. Take a 'time out' and ask the group members to discuss individual responsibilities to the group in terms of participation.
3. A possible script of questions to get a clinical problem + clinical article session going:
   - How should we manage this clinical problem?
   - What was there about the clinical article that supports that clinical decision (if unanimous) or those different decisions (if group members disagree on management)?
   - (At this point it often becomes clear that some, and maybe all, group members haven't read the article). Does anybody need time to scan the article? (If so, you may want to give them 5 minutes to see what they can glean from it.) Alternatively, you could ask them to identify the features of an article that would be most helpful to them, then assign paragraphs of the methods section to pairs of learners and have them report back to the group on how well the article met their information needs.
   - In the subsequent discussion, tease out and label the critical appraisal guides (emphasizing their generic importance rather than just how well they were met by the article).
   - If the group is stalled, you could give them the guides, assigning one each to pairs of group members, have them work for a few minutes in pairs and report back to the group what they concluded and how it affects their clinical decision.
   - What can we conclude and use in our clinical practice? Everyone agree?
   - On which clinical issues did we achieve closure? On which not? See, lifelong learning is necessary!
4. Another question to foster discussion: The methods may be sound but are the results compelling? Concepts to bring out include statistical versus clinical significance, number needed to treat, etc.

E. Cures for the 'jumping around' or 'tangent' syndrome.

1. Remember that this syndrome is not always, or even usually, a disease. It regularly leads to long-lasting competencies in the areas under discussion, especially when the disparate elements are brought together by a skilled tutor.
2. Fill in the blank spaces on a blackboard (laid out with your mind's-eye framework of the relevant list of critical

appraisal guides) as the group comes up with and discusses the relevant issues. This will allow an unstructured discussion in which learners can generate criteria, points, etc. in any order that naturally arises, yet close with a coherent, ordered summary of the key guides and issues.
3. Check your watch frequently to see how the process is going. If a lot is being generated, don't worry about keeping a particular order or you'll risk stifling creativity and active learning.
4. Try to come up with 'segues' or transitional comments to tie what might appear to be tangential issues back into the clinical business at hand.

F. Capitalize on disagreements by asking for their bases in evidence or its critical appraisal. Where possible, reconcile them as arising from the application of different critical appraisal guides or from different interpretations of evidence related to the same guide. These reconciliations can be used to involve the rest of the group and to achieve closure on the particular issue.

G. When a learner asks a question directly to the tutor, allow the question to deflect onto another member of the tutorial, by pausing or by invitation. This can accomplish two things: (a) increase the group participation, and show them that they can teach each other, (b) buy time for you to think, in case the answer isn't immediately apparent to you but you don't want to admit that too soon!

Jargon

1. Explain a concept first, then label it with the jargon term. Better yet, get the group to explain the concept.
2. Ask learners who use jargon to explain the term to the rest of the group.

Finally

Remember that those learning to practice and teach EBM usually progress through two or three levels of expertise:

1. They become very good at sniffing out biases in articles (but don't yet know their consequences). They become highly critical and risk becoming entrenched nihilists.
2. They progress to being able to identify both the presence and direction of bias, so that they can sort out whether it's tending to produce false-positive or false-negative conclusions (and can be reassured when the latter makes a positive conclusion even more, rather than less, clinically relevant). They are ready for at least intuitive sensitivity analyses. You'd like your learners to get at least this far by the end of their training.

3. They progress further and suggest (or want to learn about) ways in which the study that produced the flawed evidence could have been designed or executed that would have prevented or overcome the bias. These learners may become interested in pursuing additional education in applied research methods and should be nurtured like other budding scientists (recognizing that their colleagues may not want to pursue these methodological discussions as part of the clinical discussions).

3. The main part of the journal club session is spent in a *discussion critically appraising the evidence* found in response to the clinical problem the club identified two sessions ago (we'll call it problem A) and about which it selected evidence for detailed study one session ago. The evidence is critically appraised for its validity and applicability and a decision made about whether and how it could be applied to future patients cared for by members of the journal club. This is the 'pay-off' part of the session and every effort should be made to ensure that 'closure' is reached. Ideally, a CAT is generated along the way, for discussion, revision and distribution to all the journal club members.

The actual order of these three parts of the journal club meeting could be reversed, depending on local preferences and tardiness!

Grand rounds and clinical conferences

Most hospitals hold weekly sessions in the auditorium for either their entire clinical staff or one of its departments. These sessions, which go by *different names in different places*, are conducted in order to discuss health issues of common interest and to try to accomplish continuing education and continuing professional development. They vary enormously in their subject matter (from molecular medicine to health reform) and in the passivity of their audience and in many hospitals patients have long since disappeared from the scene.

A common thread is the attempt to instruct the audience and transfer facts to them. Alas, as we learned back in the

Introduction, such instructional forms of CME, although they may increase knowledge, don't on average bring about either useful changes in clinical behavior or improvements in the quality of care.

Could a return to the grand round of a former era improve the situation? Building on that tradition and emphasizing some principles of EBM, these meetings could take on a different flavor and convert the audience from passive to active mode. The tactics are the following:

1. The rounds begin by focusing on a specific individual patient in the care of the presenters and the patient (whenever possible), images of the patient and undigested clinical data about the patient are presented.

2. The audience are required to assess this evidence, to generate opinions on its normalcy and diagnostic, prognostic or therapeutic implications and to report their individual opinions to the assembly by show of hands. To eliminate embarrassment and encourage participation, this reporting can be done anonymously by ticking diagnostic forms and then executing two or three exchanges among neighbors so that subsequent shows of hands are known not to represent the reporter's own opinion.* Of course, this solution is unnecessary in lecture halls equipped with anonymous, keypad voting systems.

3. A critical appraisal of the relevant evidence on the diagnostic, management or other issues raised by the case is presented in an interactive fashion, requiring the audience to offer opinions on its validity and applicability.

4. A hand-out is provided at the end of the round, summarizing both the relevant evidence and the critical appraisal guides for determining its validity and clinical applicability.

In this fashion, an actively participating audience not only take stands on the appropriate evaluation and management of a real patient, but also receive a carry-away reinforcement

* It works! The author has used this approach over 100 times, with clinical audiences from five continents, and reckons that it produces participation rates of over 80%. A videotape of such a round (*Clinical Disagreement about a Patient with Dysphagia*) is available from the Centre for Evidence-Based Medicine in Oxford.

and set of guides that they can apply in other, similar situations.

Lectures (for preclinical students and clinicians of all ages and stages)

This entry may appear to be out of place! How could lectures, especially for preclinical students with no clinical skills or clinical judgment, focus in an active, interactive fashion on the care of individual patients? Well, they can, based on two realizations. First, even first year premedical students already have life experiences of a wide array of illnesses: all fear contracting AIDS, most have a relative with symptomatic coronary heart disease and many know someone with breast cancer. On the first day of school, they possess an array of personal clinical examples from which to consider the entire range of EBM topics. Second, there are unorthodox ways of employing lecture halls filled with students in ways that encourage active learning around EBM. This is perhaps best introduced by an example and the one that we will employ is a lecture to a first-year premedical class in biostatistics and epidemiology at Oxford.*

1. A clinical scenario is presented (on overheads), describing the clinical history and physical examination of a patient the speaker was called to see in an emergency room (in brief, a man who smells of alcohol and feces comes in complaining of a rapidly enlarging abdomen).

2. The students are asked to form pairs and write down the two most important facts they've been given about the patient and the two most likely explanations for his presentation. The lecturer then leaves the room for 5 minutes.

3. On return (to the sound of 60 active discussions!), the students report back their judgments and it quickly becomes apparent that there is remarkable preclinical consensus on what are considered 'clinical' issues of diagnosis.

* A videotape of this lecture (*A Stercoraceous Man with a Swollen Abdomen*) is available from the Centre for Evidence-Based Medicine in Oxford.

4. The students are then asked to identify the next most useful bit of evidence about their diagnostic explanations and the ensuing discussion around the precision and accuracy of clinical signs and symptoms introduces sensitivity, specificity, pre- and post-test probabilities, likelihood ratios and the like for later use by the faculty teaching the rest of the course.

5. Once the diagnosis and initial treatment are discussed, the issue of long-term management arises and a journal article reporting a randomized trial is distributed. Students are asked to form quartets in order to take and defend stands on whether the treatment advocated in this report should be offered to the patient. The lecturer then leaves the room for 10 minutes.

6. On return (to the roar of 30 therapeutic debates!), the students again report back their judgments and why they've decided to accept or reject the therapeutic recommendations in the published paper. The discussion introduces another host of methodological topics around descriptive and inferential statistics, statistical significance, clinically useful measures of efficacy and other topics for later use by the faculty throughout the rest of the course.

The other teachers in this course kept coming back to this patient example as they introduced the principles and methods of epidemiology and biostatistics. The students reported (in addition to enjoyment) the growing realization of the manifest relevance of understanding some epidemiological and biostatistical methodology to their goals of becoming effective clinicians.

Workshops on how to practice EBM

Although clinical learners can and do acquire the skills and knowledge for practicing EBM 'on the job' as they proceed through their careers (and this is the only site where they learn how to integrate external evidence with individual clinical expertise and apply the synthesis to patients), many learners also seek opportunities for more concentrated and focused education in its critical appraisal components. For the last 15 years, such opportunities have been provided in the form of workshops of a few hours' to a few days' duration. Originated at McMaster University in Canada, the workshop format has spread to other centers and countries and has been organized by various academic and professional groups, including a group of UK medical students who, impatient with the pace of change in undergraduate medical education, organized and ran their own 5-day workshop!* These workshops have four elements in common.

First, the learning is problem based and is typically centered around clinical scenarios describing actual patients who have been in the care of one of the faculty, accompanied by relevant research evidence (usually from the clinical literature), and calling for the learners to generate and answer questions about the clinical situation. Initially, the external evidence is provided, but later it may be the result of searches performed by the participants. By the end of the workshop, the participants will be expected to begin to pose their own questions about their own patients. An example of a clinical scenario with its citation appears in Table 4.6.3 and similar 'packages' are prepared for each of the disciplines (medicine, surgery, general practice, etc.), addressing issues in diagnosis, prognosis, therapy, systematic reviews, harm, economic analysis and quality of care.

Second, learning tends to occur in small groups of 5–10 participants with one or two tutors/facilitators who are skilled in teaching EBM and in running small groups. This provides an environment that encourages active learning and often replicates the clinical team settings in which EBM will be practiced subsequently. While carefully avoiding behavioral therapy, these groups also instruct and encourage their members in more effective and efficient team function by developing and following rules such as those that appear in Table 4.6.4. Each group meeting begins by setting an agenda for the session (including setting aside time for breaks, evaluation, future planning); agreeing on the clinical problem, the roles of group members, the educational tasks and the evidence to be appraised; getting on with it (calling 'time out' when either the process or the content is getting bogged down); evaluating this session;

* Named OCCAMS for Oxford Conference on Critical Appraisal for Medical Students and involving students from England, Scotland, Northern Ireland, Germany, Sweden and Croatia.

Table 4.6.3 A clinical scenario to initiate problem-based learning around an issue in therapy

You learn that a 54 y/o man with NIDDM (on oral hypoglycemics) whose myocardial infarction you treated 6 months ago has died suddenly at home. Wondering whether you could have done more for him, you review his notes and confirm that his was, in fact, a low-risk inferior MI with no complications whose blood sugar was elevated on admission (13 mmol/L) but settled down within 3 days.

In view of the success of 'tight control' of IDDM in preventing or postponing retinopathy and neuropathy, you wonder if a more aggressive treatment of his NIDDM might have postponed his untimely death. On the other hand, you well recall how one of your Profs back in medical school insisted that insulin was atherogenic and how you should back off insulin doses when diabetics developed angina pectoris.

So you form the clinical question: 'Among patients with NIDDM who are having MIs, does tight control of their blood sugar reduce their risk of dying?'

On your own or with help from the librarian at your local postgraduate center, you find the attached article: Malmberg K et al Randomized trial of insulin-glucose infusion followed by subcutaneous insulin treatment in diabetic patients with acute myocardial infarction (DIGAMI Study). J Am Coll Cardiol 1995; 26: 57–65.*

Read it (to possibly help you, we've included bits of a book on how to read clinical articles) and decide:
1. whether it answers your question;
2. if so, what the answer is;
whether you and your hospital colleagues should review how you are treating diabetic patients with myocardial infarctions.

* It can also be found on the disk version of *ACP Journal Club/Evidence-Based Medicine* or via MEDLINE using the terms: diabetes mellitus AND myocardial infarction AND publication type=randomized controlled trial.

Table 4.6.4 How small groups succeed in learning EBM (or anything else)

1. **By taking responsibility (individually and as a group) for showing up and on time; by learning each other's names, interests and objectives; by respecting each other; by contributing to, accepting and supporting individual and group rules of behavior, including confidentiality; by contributing to, accepting and supporting both the overall objectives of the group and the detailed plans and assignments for each session; by carrying out the agreed plans and assignments, including role playing; by listening (concentrating and analyzing, rather than simply preparing your own response to what's being said) and by talking (including consolidating and summarizing).**
2. **By monitoring and (by using time in/time out*) reinforcing positive and correcting negative elements of both:**
   - **'process', regarding educational methods (reinforcing positive contributions and teaching methods; proposing strategies for improving less effective ones) and responsibility (identifying behaviors, not motives; encouraging [e.g. with eye-contact, verbally] non-participants; quieting down [e.g. move them next to tutor] overparticipants); and**
   - **'content': unclear, uncertain or incorrect facts or critical appraisal principles/ strategies/ tactics.**
3. **By evaluating selves, each other, the group, the session and the program with candour and respect, 'celebrating' what went well (and should be preserved) and identifying what went poorly, focusing on strategies for correcting/ improving the situation.**

* Time in for the teaching/learning portions of the session, especially when using role play, time out for discussions of effective/ineffective teaching/learning methods and group/individual behavior.

and planning for the next one. Thus, the learning focuses on the five steps that form the major chapters of this book:

1. forming answerable questions;
2. searching for the best evidence (workshops usually include individual tutorials by librarians experienced in teaching searching skills);
3. critically appraising the evidence (the major focus of most workshops);

4. integrating the appraisal with individual clinical expertise and applying it in practice (this element can only be carried out when workshops are spread out over longer periods of time, with regular clinical responsibilities taking place between sessions); and
5. self-evaluation.

Given the foregoing, the selection of participants (in addition to responding to consumer demand and general interest) seeks individuals who are already receptive to EBM (skeptics make important contributions to workshops and are welcome additions to the converted) and are likely to be able to apply what they learn in their clinical practice. Most evaluations suggest that small groups made up of clinicians in the same discipline (e.g. general practice, surgery, nursing, etc.) learn best, as they can work on scenarios specific to their disciplines and more readily see how they might apply the results of their growing skills in practice. The exceptions to this rule are methodologists such as epidemiologists and biostatisticians, who are often used to functioning in disparate groups and can contribute to one of any make-up. The play of chance and small numbers (surgical specialities often are underrepresented) sometimes makes for unusual combinations of disciplines and these often require additional attention to be sure that alternative scenarios are presented to maintain relevance for all members.

Third, lots of time is set aside for small group meetings, individual study and meetings of ad hoc interest groups. Educational materials are sent out well in advance (with a reassurance that not all have to be mastered before the workshop!). A typical schedule is shown in Table 4.6.5. Tutors meet daily to report progress, to make mid-course corrections in the workshop and to identify and solve problems in group function and learning (their training occurs in the 'how to teach EBM' workshops described in Chapter 5). Plenary sessions are kept to a minimum and deal only with issues best communicated in a lecture or lecture-audience participation format (a review of EBM, how to pose answerable questions, an introduction to information searching, etc.) and a final feedback and evaluation session where par-

Table 4.6.5 A typical schedule for a workshop on how to practice EBM

Time	Sunday	Monday	Tuesday	Wednesday	Thursday	Friday
0800		Tutors' meetings				
0900		Plenary sessions on forming questions, searching, etc.				Small groups
1000		Small groups	Small groups	Small groups	Small groups	
1100						Evaluation
1200		Lunch				Good-bye
1300		Individual study or ad hoc interest group meetings or individual searching				
1400	Tutors' meeting					
1500						
1600	Small groups	Small groups	Small groups	Small groups	Small groups	
1700						
1800	Supper					
Evening	Social	Study	Social	Study	Social	

ticipants hand in their evaluation forms and suggest improvements for future workshops.

Some workshops are held in one-day or half-day sessions, spread out over longer periods of time. Less efficient for organizers, these often merge with the journal clubs described above and provide more opportunities for integrating the critical appraisals with individual clinical expertise as the EBM skills are acquired.

Fourth, participants and organizers keep in touch after the workshops in order to continue to trade ideas on how to practice EBM, how to improve future workshops and so that some of the participants can move to the next level of not only practicing EBM but teaching it as well. These workshops will be described in Chapter 5.

Further information

Get on the WWW and browse the educational resources of the Centre for Evidence-Based Medicine in Oxford by contacting the Uniform Resource Locator: http://cebm.jr2.ox.ac.uk/

Individuals interested in attending or organizing workshops in how to practise EBM can contact either the Department of Clinical Epidemiology and Biostatistics at McMaster University (1200 Main Street West, Hamilton, Ontario, Canada L8N 3Z5) or any of the Centres for Evidence-Based Practice in the UK (for example: http://cebm.jr2.ox.ac.uk/ will get you to the Website for the Centre for Evidence-Based Medicine in Oxford).

(Prepared for this book by Douglas G. Altman of the ICRF Medical Statistics Group and the Centre for Statistics in Medicine, Oxford, UK)

What does the 'confidence interval', abbreviated CI, tell us? The CI gives a measure of the precision (or uncertainty) of study results for making inferences about the population of all such patients. A strictly correct definition of a 95% CI is, somewhat opaquely, that 95% of such intervals will contain the true population value. Little is lost by the less pure interpretation of the CI as the range of values within which we can be 95% sure that the population value lies. The CI approach places a clear emphasis on quantification, in direct contrast to the P values which arise from the significance testing approach. The P value is not an estimate of any quantity but rather a measure of the strength of evidence against the null hypothesis of 'no effect'. The P value by itself tells us nothing about the size of a difference, nor even the direction of that difference. P values on their own are thus not informative in papers or abstracts. By contrast, CIs indicate the strength of evidence about quantities of direct interest, such as treatment benefit. They are thus of particular relevance to practitioners of evidence-based medicine.[1-3]

The estimation approach to statistical analysis exemplified in the CI aims to quantify the effect of interest (the sensitivity of a diagnostic test, the rate of a prognostic event, the NNT for a treatment, etc.) and also to quantify the uncertainty in this effect. Most often this is a range of values either side of the estimate in which we can be 95% sure that the true value lies. The convention of using the value of 95% is arbitrary, just as is that of taking $P < 0.05$ as being significant, and authors sometimes use 90% or 99% CIs. Note that the word 'interval' means a range of values and is thus singular. The two values that define the interval are called 'confidence limits'.

The CI is based on the idea that the same study carried out on different samples of patients would not yield identical results, but would be spread around the true but unknown result. The CI estimates this 'sampling variation'. In most circumstances the CI is calculated from the observed estimate of the quantity of interest, such as the difference (d) between two proportions, and the standard error (SE) of the estimate for this difference. A 95% CI is obtained here as $d \pm 1.96SE$ (the formula will vary according to the nature of the outcome measure and the coverage of the CI, but it will be of this general type). Table A.1 gives the structure of the SEs for some clinical measurements of interest. For example, in a randomized placebo-controlled trial of acellular pertussis vaccine,[4] 72/1670 (4.3%) infants developed pertussis among those receiving the vaccine and 240/1665 (14.4%) did so among the control group. The difference in percentages, known as the absolute risk reduction, is 10.1%. The SE of this difference is 0.99%, so that the 95% CI is 10.1% ± 1.96 × 0.99% and therefore runs from 8.2% to 12.0%.

Despite the considerably different philosophical approaches CIs and significance tests are closely related mathematically. Thus a 'significant' P value of $P < 0.05$ will correspond to a 95% CI which excludes the value indicating equality; for example, this value is 0 for the difference between two means or proportions and 1 for a relative risk or odds ratio. (The equivalence of the two approaches may not be exact in some circumstances.) The prevailing view is that estimation, including CIs, is the preferable approach to summarizing the results of a study, but CIs and P values are complementary and many papers use both.

The uncertainty (imprecision) expressed by a CI is to a large extent affected by the square root of the sample size. Small samples provide less information than large ones and the CI is correspondingly wider in a smaller sample. For example, a paper comparing the characteristics of three tests to diagnose *H. pylori*[5] reported the sensitivity of the ^{14}C urea breath test as 95.8% (95% CI 75% to 100%). While the figure of 95.8% is impressive, the small sample of 24 adults with *H. pylori* means that there is considerable uncertainty in that estimate as shown by the wide CI. If the same sensitivity had been observed in a sample of 240, the 95% CI would have been from 92.5% to 98.0%.

Table A.1 Standard errors (SEs) and confidence intervals (CIs) for some clinical measures of interest

Clinical measure	Standard error (SE)	Typical calculation of SE and CI
(a) When the outcome is an event – one group		
Proportion (as in Sensitivity, Event Rate, etc.)	$SE = \sqrt{\frac{p \times (1-p)}{n}}$ where p is proportion and n is number of patients	If p=24/60=0.4 (or 40%): $SE = \sqrt{\frac{0.4 \times 0.6}{60}} = 0.063$ (or 6.3%) 95% CI is 40% ± 1.96 × 6.3% or 27.6% to 52.4%
*(b) When the outcome is an event – comparison of two groups**		
In general, r_1 and r_2 events are observed among n_1 and n_2 patients in two groups, so the observed proportions are $p_1=r_1/n_1$ and $p_2=r_2/n_2$. In the illustrative example, $p_1=15/125$ (or 12%) and $p_2=30/120=0.25$ (or 25%).		
Absolute Risk Reduction (ARR)	$SE = \sqrt{\frac{p_1(1-p_1)}{n_1} + \frac{p_2(1-p_2)}{n_2}}$	$ARR = p_2 - p_1 = 0.13$ (or 13%): $SE = \sqrt{\frac{0.12 \times 0.88}{125} + \frac{0.25 \times 0.75}{120}} = 0.049$ (or 4.9%) **95% CI is 13% ± 1.96 × 4.9%, i.e. 3.4% to 22.6%**

Number Needed to Treat (NNT)	**Not calculated**	**NNT=100/ARR=100/13=7.7; CI is obtained as reciprocal of CI for ARR, so 95% CI is 100/22.6 to 100/3.4 or 4.4 to 29.4**
Relative Risk (RR)	$RR=p_1/p_2$ SE of log (RR) = $\sqrt{\frac{1}{r_1}+\frac{1}{r_2}-\frac{1}{n_1}-\frac{1}{n_2}}$	RR=0.12/0.25=0.48 (48%); log (RR)=-0.734; SE of log(RR) = $\sqrt{\frac{1}{15}+\frac{1}{30}-\frac{1}{125}-\frac{1}{120}}=0.289$; 95% CI for log(RR) is −0.734±1.96×0.289, i.e. −1.301 to −0.167; 95% CI for RR is 0.272 to 0.846 or 27.2% to 84.6%.
Relative Risk Reduction (RRR)	Not calculated	$RRR=1-RR=1-p_2/p_1=1-12/25=0.52$ (or 52%). 95% CI for RRR is obtained by subtracting CI for RR from 1 (or 100%), i.e. 0.154 to 0.728 or 15.4% to 72.8%
Odds ratio (OR)	$OR=\frac{r_1(n_2-r_2)}{r_2(n_1-n_1)}$ SE of log(OR) $=\sqrt{\frac{1}{r_1}+\frac{1}{r_2}+\frac{1}{n_1-r_1}+\frac{1}{n_2-r_2}}$	$OR=\frac{15\times90}{30\times110}=0.409$; log(OR)=-0.894 SE of log(OR) = $\sqrt{\frac{1}{15}+\frac{1}{30}+\frac{1}{90}+\frac{1}{110}}=0.347$ 95% CI for log(OR) is -0.894±1.96×0.347, or -1.573 to -0.214; 95% CI for OR is 0.207 to 0.807.

Table A.1 *continued.*

Clinical measure	Standard error (SE)	Typical calculation of SE and CI
(c) When the outcome is a continuous measurement		
Mean	If s is standard deviation (SD) of n observations, $SE=s/\sqrt{n}$	95% CI is mean ±t ×SE (see footnote 2). If mean =17.2, s=6.4, n=38, then $SE=6.4/\sqrt{38}=1.038$ and 95% CI is 17.2±2.026×1.038 or 15.1 to 19.3
Difference between two means	If s_1 and s_2 are SDs of n_1 and n_2 observations, SE(diff) = $\sqrt{\frac{(n_1-1)s_1^2+(n_2-1)s_2^2}{n_1+n_2-2}\times\left(\frac{1}{n_1}+\frac{1}{n_2}\right)}$	95% CI is mean diff±t×SE(diff) (see footnote 2). If $mean_1=17.2$, $s_1=6.4$, $n_1=38$, $mean_2=15.9$, $s_2=5.6$, $n_2=45$, then mean difference=d=17.2−15.9=1.3, $SE(diff)=\sqrt{\frac{37\times6.4^2+44\times5.6^2}{38+45-2}\times\left(\frac{1}{38}+\frac{1}{45}\right)}=1.317$ **and 95% CI is 1.3±1.99×1.317 or -1.32 to 3.92.**

1. In general a confidence interval is obtained by taking the estimate of interest and adding and subtracting a multiple of the SE. Except in the case of means or differences in means, the multiple is taken as a value from the standard normal distribution. For a 95% CI the multiplier is 1.96; for a 90% CI it is 1.645, and for a 99% CI it is 2.576. For RR (and RRR) and OR the CI is obtained for the logarithm of the quantity of interest and antilogged (logs to base e are used in the Table).
2. The calculation of a CI for a mean or the difference between means the multiplier for a 95% CI is not 1.96 but a value from the t distribution with n−1 or n_1+n_2-2 degrees of freedom (df) respectively. For df larger than 40 this value is close to 2.
3. The above calculations assume that comparisons are between two independent groups. For CIs derived from paired data (e.g. from crossover trials or matched case-control studies), and also CIs for some other statistics, see Gardner MJ and Altman DG (eds) Statistics with confidence. London: BMJ, 1989.
* As used in this book, p_1 corresponds to the event rate in the experimental group (EER) and p_2 to the event rate in the control group (CER).

Non-significant results in randomized trials (i.e. those with P > 0.05) are especially prone to misinterpretation. CIs are especially useful here as they show whether the data are compatible with clinically useful true effects. For example, one of the outcomes in a randomized trial to compare suturing and stapling for large-bowel anastomosis[6] was wound infection, which occurred in 10.9% and 13.5% of cases respectively (P=0.30). The 95% CI for this difference of 2.6% is −2% to +8%. Even in this study of 652 patients there thus remains the possibility that there is a modest difference in wound infection rates for the two procedures. In a smaller study, uncertainty is greater. Sung et al[7] carried out a randomized trial to compare octreotide infusion and emergency sclerotherapy for acute variceal hemorrhage in 100 patients. The observed rates of controlled bleeding were 84% in the octreotide group and 90% in the sclerotherapy group, giving P=0.56. Note that the figures for uncontrolled bleeding are similar to those for wound infection in the study just considered. In this case, however, the 95% CI for the treatment difference of 6% is −7% to +19%. This interval is very wide in relation to the 5% difference that was of interest. It is clear that the study cannot rule out a large difference in effectiveness, so that the authors' conclusion that 'octreotide infusion and sclerotherapy are equally effective in controlling variceal hemorrhage' is certainly not valid.

CIs can be constructed for most common statistical estimates or comparisons.[8] For RCTs, these include differences between means or proportions, relative risks, odds ratios and the number needed to treat (NNT). A computer program for personal computers which covers many of these methods is available from the *British Medical Journal*.[9] Likewise, CIs can be obtained for all the main estimates arising in studies of diagnosis – sensitivity, specificity, positive predictive value (all of which are simple proportions) – and estimates derived from metaanalyses and case-control studies.

While CIs are desirable for the primary results of a study, they are not needed for all results. Further, it is important that when given, they relate to the contrast of interest. In particular, when two groups are compared the appropriate CI is that for the difference between the groups, as illustrated in the above examples. Not only is it unhelpful to give separate CIs for the estimates in each group, but this presentation can be quite misleading. When the authors have not provided CIs, these can often be constructed using the results provided in their paper.

The most appropriate methods of statistical analysis and presentation must be largely a matter for personal judgment, although increasingly journals are requesting or requiring authors to use CIs when presenting their key findings. It seems clear that the wide adoption of CIs in medical research papers over the last decade has been of great benefit to a more correct understanding of the external evidence used in the practice of evidence-based medicine.

References

1 Gardner M J, Altman D G. Confidence intervals rather than P values: estimation rather than hypothesis testing. BMJ 1986; 292: 746–50.

2 Rothman K J, Yankauer A. Confidence intervals vs. significance tests: quantitative interpretation. Am J Public Health 1986; 76.587–8.

3 Bulpitt C J. Confidence intervals. Lancet 1986; 1: 494–7.

4 Trollfors B et al. A placebo-controlled trial of a pertussis-toxoid vaccine. N Eng J Med 1995; 333: 1045–50.

5 Fallone C A et al. Determination of test performance of less costly methods of *Helicobacter pylori* detection. Clin Invest Med 1995; 18: 177–85.

6 Docherty J G et al. Comparison of manually constructed and stapled anastomoses in colorectal surgery. Ann Surg, 1995; 221: 176–84.

7 Sung J J Y, Chung S C S, Lai C-W et al. Octreotide infusion or emergency sclerotherapy for variceal haemorrhage. Lancet 1993; 342: 637–41.

8 Gardner M J, Altman D G (eds). Statistics with confidence. British Medical Journal, London, 1989.

9 Gardner M J, Gardner S B, Winter P D. Confidence interval analysis (CIA) microcomputer program manual. British Medical Journal, London, 1989.

The educational materials for each session include:

1 A clinical scenario based on a real patient we've seen on our service.
2 The clinical question that arose from caring for this patient.
3 The searching strategy we employed in looking for external evidence.
4 The results of that search.
5 A description of the skills-training elements of Part B of the session.
6 A blank worksheet of users' guides for critically appraising that evidence for its validity and potential clinical usefulness.
7 A completed worksheet, showing what we thought of it – the answers might not be right, but they're ours! This is for the benefit of those who are teaching the course and for the evaluation purposes, so they can be separated from the pre-circulated materials and saved for later on.
8 A CAT summarising the article. Again, thse can be separated from the pre-circulated materials.

Note: Learners' packs have items 1–6 separated from items 7–8.

If you aren't familiar with teaching EBCH, you might want to attend one of the short courses on *How to practise evidence-based child health* that are held at various locations each year. These courses aim to help practitioners use the best available evidence in their clinical and policy decisions. The course consists of plenary seminars, small group problem-solving and appraisal sessions based on clinical and policy scenarios in child health, and practical sessions on how to search the scientific literature. To find out when and where the next short course is being held, look on our web page: **http://www.ich.ucl.ac.uk/ebm/ebm.htm** or email: **cebch@ich.ucl.ac.uk**

Several of the teaching methods that can be used in this course are described on pp 188–97 of *Evidence-based Medicine: how to practice and teach EBM,* by D Sackett, W Richardson, W Rosenberg, and R Haynes (published by Churchill-Livingstone). Pages from *Evidence-based Medicine,* referred to in the sessions, are produced in full at the back of this manual.

There are several different ways to lead the discussions of the clinical scenarios and papers in these sessions:

1 We suggest that you begin all of them by being sure that the learners understand the patient's biological and clinical problem and the 3- (or 4-) part clinical question.
2 The objective is to help the learners apply the users' guides to this paper and understand them well enough to be able to apply them to subsequent simpler papers. You can accomplish this in different ways:
   – you could ask the group (either all together or in groups of two to four) to apply each of the guides in turn, and discuss them and their application in sequence. This approach is more efficient but less self-directed, and is useful when time is scarce or the group is reticent about expressing their views

- at the other extreme, you could initiate a free-form discussion by asking learners to take and defend their stands on whether they would apply the paper's conclusions to the patient, and then draw the guides out of this discussion. The approach encourages self-directed learning, but is less efficient than the tutor-directed approach and requires a group who is comfortable expressing their views.

3 At the end you could hand out the completed worksheets and CATs.

4 We urge you to end each session by evaluating it with the learners, identifying ways that they, you and the readings could be improved for the next time.

To run this course, we borrow heavily from the expertise and resources developed by the Evidence-Based Medicine working group. Resources include:

1 Two of our local librarians – John Clarke and Reinhard Wentz – who run the session on searching and have developed a teaching package for undergraduate and graduate learners. They are members of the Centre and can be contacted through the Centre for Evidence-Based Child Health. Alternatively, contact the Centre for Evidence-Based Child Health for additional information from Robin Snowball, who runs the search sessions for the Evidence-Based Medicine training.

2 Reference to the book and the cards inside it – these pages are colour-coded to match the relevant cards. *Evidence-based Medicine: how to practice and teach EBM,* by D Sackett, W Richardson, W Rosenberg, and R Haynes (published by Churchill-Livingstone). You may already have another reference with which you're more familiar or find more useful.

3 For you and your learners to make optimal use of this syllabus you and they will need easy access to computers that include both CD-ROM and Internet access.

4 *Best Evidence,* a CD with cumulated abstracts and other materials from *ACP Journal Club* and *Evidence-based Medicine,* two journals of critically appraised articles from an array of clinical journals covering internal medicine, general practice, obstetrics and gynaecology, paediatrics, psychiatry and surgery. This resource can be ordered from the BMJ Publishing Group (PO Box 295, London WC1H 9TE; Tel: 0171 387 4499 and ask for 'Subscriptions'; Fax: 0171 383 6662; e-mail: bmjsubs@dial.pipex.com).

5 One of the MEDLINE searching systems (we used *WinSPIRS*). Members of the British Medical Association can obtain 'quick searches' and access MEDLINE (via modem or Internet) at no charge (to sign up, call BMA Library at 0171 383 6625).

6 CATMaker, a software program developed for analysing, summarising and storing critical appraisals. It can be obtained from the Evidence-Based Medicine Centre in Oxford and from their website.

7 The Centre for Evidence-based Medicine's website (**http://cebm.jr2.ox.ac.uk**) where several banks of clinically useful measures on the precision and accuracy of clinical exam and lab test results (SpPins, SnNouts, sensitivities, specificities, likelihood ratios), on the power of prognostic factors, and therapy (NNTs, RRRs and the like) can be found.

8 For demonstrating *Best Evidence,* MEDLINE searching, the CATMaker, and our website, we used a computer projector device that displayed the contents of a computer screen onto the wall for all to see. In our sessions, half are doctors.

   This program is suitable for a mixed group of paediatricians, GPs, nurses, health visitors, physiotherapists, speech therapists and managers, etc.

   The scenarios and papers in this particular package have been designed for tutors and trainees whose work relates to child health, however, they could easily be replaced by ones more appropriate for general practice or other specialities.

If you wish to teach with this package, additional copies can be obtained from our Centre. They are of two sorts

1 Tutors' packages: like this one, containing all the materials for the course.
2 Learners' packages:
   - have the complete set of course materials but the completed worksheets and CATs will be separated from each scenario;
   - tutors' notes are not included.

We look forward to receiving feedback and suggestions for how we might improve this course.

And if you have any similar educational resource materials that you would like to announce on our website, please contact us.

Maud Meates
Olivier Duperrex
Ruth Gilbert
Stuart Logan
Centre for Evidence-Based Child Health

EBCH SESSION

1

TUTOR'S GUIDE

Therapy and introduction to CATS

This session on intervention provides three options:

1. A scenario involving setting up a nurse-led education programme to reduce asthma readmissions.
2. A scenario about whether to modify a postal reminder to improve immunisation rates.
3. A scenario involving treatment of a child with mild croup.

All three examples show how to obtain a number needed to treat (NNT) for your population. The postal reminder paper has a good discussion regarding 'intention to treat' and may be more suitable for beginners. All three articles will generate discussion about applicability.

The study on croup is good for beginners and, for more advanced students, raises the question of whether the relative risk can be applied to similar children seen in primary care.

We've provided three complete sets of handouts for the alternative patients.

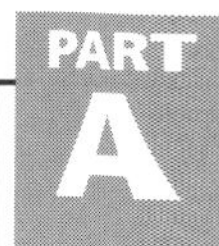

Critical appraisal of a clinical article about therapy (suggested minimum time allotment: 60 minutes)

EBCH SESSION

1

TUTOR'S GUIDE

SECTIONS 1,2,3

Therapy and introduction to CATs

Learning objectives

1. **To introduce the concept of critical appraisal and the use of critical appraisal guides and worksheets.**
2. **To learn how to critically appraise evidence about therapy for its validity, importance and usefulness.**
3. **To introduce the number needed to treat (NNT) as a clinically useful measure that can be derived from research reports.**
4. **To stress the application of research evidence to the individual patient.**

There are several different ways to lead the discussion of this and the subsequent four sessions (they are discussed in greater detail on pp 188–97 *Evidence-based Medicine*):

1. We suggest that you begin all of them by ensuring that the learners understand the patient's biological and clinical problem and the 3- (or 4-) part clinical question.
2. The ultimate objective is to help the learners apply the users' guides to this paper and understand them well enough to apply them to subsequent papers about therapy. You can accomplish this in different ways:
   - You could ask them (either all together or in groups of two to four) to apply each of the guides in turn, and discuss them and their application in sequence. This approach is more efficient but less self-directed, and is useful when time is scarce or the group is reticent about expressing their views.
   - At the other extreme, you could initiate a free-form discussion by asking learners to take and defend their stands on whether they would apply the paper's conclusions to the patient, and then draw the guides out of this discussion. This approach encourages self-directed learning, but is less efficient than the tutor-directed approach and requires a group who is expressing their views.
3. At the end you could hand out the completed worksheets and CATs.
4. We urge you to end each session by evaluating it with the learners, identifying ways that they, you and the readings could be improved for next time.

EBCH SESSION

6

TUTOR'S GUIDE

Presentations and searching the Cochrane Library

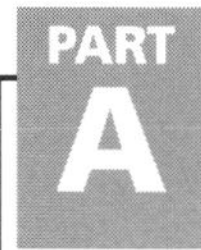

PART A Presentations

Depending on the number of learners who are presenting their own cases, you may find that you require just one session for these (and for the introduction to the Cochrane Library). In that case, you can either shorten the course to 6 sessions or give them one 'open' session in which they can come to you for advice and help with searching for, critically appraising, or summarising their evidence, or to raise other issues in critical appraisal, EBM generally, etc.

PART B Searching the Cochrane Library (suggested minimum time allotment: 30 minutes)

Learning objectives

1. **To learn how to look for evidence in the Cochrane Library, including:**
   - **Cochrane Reviews**
   - **DARE (the Database of Abstracts of Reviews of Effectiveness)**
   - **the clinical trials registry.**
2. **To gain information about the Cochrane Collaboration (and encouragement to join it!)**

In demonstrating the Cochrane Library, you might want to have done enough homework to have identified some systematic reviews that are of great relevance to your learners.

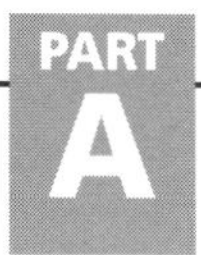

PART A Presentations

The other half of the participants will present their patients, questions, critically appraised topics, and clinical conclusions.

Presentations, feedback and celebration

PART B Feedback and celebration

Learning objectives

1. **To evaluate the course ('Evaluation of 'practising EBCH'') in order to:**
   - **improve it for the next time you give it**
   - **provide feedback to the developers of this course back in Oxford.**
2. **To permit the learners to evaluate their own performance ('Am I Practising EBCH?')**
3. **To decide where you and the learners want to go from here in continuing to learn and practise EBCH (e.g. the clinical rounds, academic half-days, journal clubs, etc. described on pp 185–206 of *Evidence-based Medicine*).**

The final portion of the session (and course!) can be spent evaluating the course. The attached forms permit written feedback, and a discussion will be held on general issues.

We'd urge you to devote special attention to discussing and deciding what to do with what has been learned, and how to continue to improve and use this set of clinical, EBM and self-directed learning skills on clinical rounds, in academic half-days, journal clubs, etc.